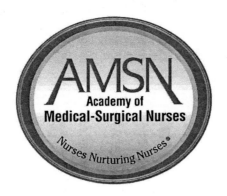

Medical-Surgical Nursing
Review Questions

© Copyright 2008
2nd Edition
Academy of Medical-Surgical Nurses
East Holly Avenue/Box 56, Pitman, NJ 08071-0056
Phone: 866-877-AMSN (2676)
Fax: 856-589-7463
E-mail: amsn@ajj.com
Web site: www.medsurgnurse.org
ISBN: 978-0-9795029-5-8

Publication Management by Anthony J. Jannetti, Inc.
East Holly Avenue/Box 56, Pitman, NJ 08071-0056

Medical-Surgical Nursing Review Questions

EDITOR

Dottie Roberts, MSN, MACI, RN, CMSRN, OCNS-C
Clinical Nurse Specialist, Rehabilitative & Medical Services
Palmetto Health Baptist
Columbia, SC

ITEM WRITERS

Janice Castro, MSN, RN, CNS
Clinical Nurse Specialist
Medical-Surgical, Telemetry, and Behavioral Health
Services
Community Hospital of San Bernardino
San Bernardino, CA

Arnold deLeon, MSN, RN, CMSRN
Team Leader/4 South
George Washington University Hospital
Washington, DC

Stephanie Nicole Frost, MHA, BSN, RN-BC
Staff Nurse
Michael E. DeBakey VA Medical Center
Houston, TX

Debra Garrett, RN-C, CMSRN
Solid Organ & Stem Cell Nurse Transplant/Hospital
Nurse Consultant
North Carolina Division of Medical Assistance
Raleigh, NC

Perry Goldstein, BSN, RN, CMSRN
Nurse Case Manager
Personal Touch Home Care
Fort Thomas, KY

Wendy Goodson-Celerin, MS, ARNP, CNA-BC, CMSRN
Nurse Manager, Specialty Surgery Unit
Tampa General Hospital
Tampa, FL

Kathleen Marchiondo, MSN, RN, CMSRN
Assistant Professor
University of Central Missouri
Kansas City, MO

Tracy Sansossio, BSN, RN, CMSRN
Acute Care Coordinator
Augusta Medical Center
Fishersville, VA

Lori Shults, BSN, RN, CMSRN
Staff Nurse
Northern Nevada Medical Center
Sparks, NV

Theresa M. Smith, BSN, RN, CMSRN
Team Leader, 6SS
Miami Valley Hospital
Dayton, OH

REVIEWERS

Caroline Ashman, RN, CMSRN
Medical-Surgical Nurse
Emory East Side Hospital
Snellville, GA

Betty Jo Ernst, MSN, RN, CMSRN
Clinical Outcomes Manager for
Heart Failure
St. John's Mercy Medical Center
St. Louis, MO

Roberta Harbison, MSN, RN,
CMSRN
Medical-Surgical Nurse
Redlands, CA

Robin Hertel, BSN, RN, CMSRN
Nursing Instructor
North Central Kansas Technical
College
Hays, KS

Kathleen Marchiondo, MSN, RN,
CMSRN
Assistant Professor
Central Missouri State University
Kansas City, MO

Vicky Overby, MSN, RN, CMSRN
Clinical Nurse Specialist for
Medical-Surgical Services
Rex Healthcare
Raleigh, NC

Hope Slone, BSN, RN, CMSRN, CPAN
Staff Development Educator
Sentara Norfolk General Hospital
Norfolk, VA

Barbara Smith, MEd, RN, CEN,
CMSRN
Nurse Educator, Adult Health and
Emergency Services
St Luke's Health Care System
Boise, ID

Sharon S. Taylor, BSN, RN, CMSRN
Medical-Surgical Nurse and
Educator
Columbus Regional Hospital
Columbus, IN

Introduction

The second edition of this valuable resource will provide an excellent review for anyone who is new to the exciting world of medical-surgical nursing. This includes new graduates as well as nurses who have worked in other settings before moving to a medical-surgical unit. In reality, though, the book is most likely to be used by nurses preparing for the medical-surgical nursing specialty certification examination.

Certification, as defined by the American Board of Nursing Specialties (ABNS) (2005), is "the formal recognition of the specialized knowledge, skills, and experience demonstrated by the achievement of standards identified by a nursing specialty to promote optimal health outcomes." All nurses are required to have licensure to practice, but certification for most of them is an option pursued as an important step in professional development. Some employers honor and identify certified nurses in various ways, while others offer no recognition. To many certified nurses, the benefit of their achievement is intrinsic; they know they have demonstrated knowledge that helps them provide expert care during every shift of work.

The certification examination offered by the Medical-Surgical Nursing Certification Board (MSNCB) is based on the analysis of practice of hundreds of nurses in the specialty. Test developers identified areas of emphasis to guide the construction of exam items. In addition, a theoretical framework was paired with the analysis to further ensure the examination accurately reflects medical-surgical nursing practice. The seven domains of nurse practice identified by Patricia Benner serve as one axis for the exam content, with patient problems as the other axis. The following blueprint demonstrates these areas of emphasis for the examination:

Patient Problems by Physiologic System
Pulmonary (18% – 20% of questions)
Cardiovascular (14% – 16%)
Gastrointestinal (18% – 20%)
Genitourinary, Renal, and Reproductive (11% – 13%)
Musculoskeletal and Neurologic (10% – 12%)
Hematologic, Immunologic, and Integumentary (8% – 10%)
Diabetes and Other Endocrine (14% – 16%)

Domains of Nursing Practice*
Helping Role (16% – 18% of questions)
Teaching/Coaching Function (16% – 18%)
Diagnostic and Patient Monitoring Function (24% – 26%)
Administering/Monitoring Therapeutic Interventions (24% – 26%)
Managing Rapidly Changing Situations (9% – 11%)
Monitoring/Ensuring Quality of Health Care Practices (2% – 4%)
Organizational and Work Role Competencies (2% – 4%)

The items in this publication have been written by content experts to reflect the emphasis placed on physiological systems in the medical-surgical nursing certification exam. In addition, the items are identified based on the domains of nursing practice (see coding included with answers). They are typical of the type of questions that will be encountered by candidates for medical-surgical nursing certification. However, none of the actual examination questions is included in this publication.

All contributors to this resource are personally committed to the competent practice of medical-surgical nursing and to specialty nursing certification. Our sincere hope is that this text will help even more nurses reach the milestone of excellence demonstrated by medical-surgical certification. For those who utilize it for professional review, we trust it will enrich your practice.

Dottie Roberts, MSN, MACI, RN, CMSRN, OCNS-C
Editor

Reference

American Board of Nursing Specialties (ABNS). (2005). *A position statement on the value of specialty nursing certification.* Retrieved January 6, 2008, from http://www.nursingcertification.org/pdf/value_certification.pdf

For more information abut medical-surgical nursing certification, contact the MSNCB at East Holly Avenue/Box 56; Pitman, NJ 08071-0056 (msncb@ajj.com). The examination application is available on the AMSN Web site (www.medsurgnurse.org/cert) or through the test agency C-NET, 601 Pavonia Avenue, Suite 201, Jersey City, NJ 07306 (garbin@cnetnurse.com).

*See next page for a detailed description of the domains.

Directions for Using These Review Questions

1. Complete all multiple choice items or focus upon the items specific to one or more of the exam categories.
2. Read each multiple choice item carefully and circle your answer on the Answer Sheets provided at the end of this publication.
   - Try to answer the question before reading options.
   - Underline key words.
   - Do not read anything more into the question or options than what is there; do not over analyze.
   - If unsure of the answer, use logic to rule out options that could be correct versus those that are definitely incorrect.
   - Select options that reflect a nursing judgment.
   - If two answers appear to be correct, choose the one that causes the other to occur.
   - Select options that are correct without exception.
   - When evaluating difficult test questions, mark the options you think are wrong.
   - Avoid options that are true statements, but do not answer the question.

3. Check the correct answers using the Answer Key located at the end of this publication.
4. There is no passing score for this assessment. Reward yourself for the items you answer correctly. Review those items that you answer incorrectly to determine your areas for further study.

Disclaimer: These review questions provide an opportunity to assess your knowledge of selected components of medical-surgical nursing practice and to practice answering multiple choice items. They do not represent a comprehensive compilation of all content comprising medical-surgical nursing practice. Completion of these test questions does not guarantee the examinee will pass the certification exam. The authors and reviewers of these study questions are NOT item writers or content expert panel members for the Medical-Surgical Nursing Certification Examination offered by the Medical-Surgical Nursing Certification Board.

Domains of Medical-Surgical Nursing Practice

These seven domains of nursing practice serve as an important component of the CMSRN examination blueprint.

I. Helping Role

1. Use culturally-sensitive and age-specific instruments to assess patient's level of comfort (e.g., pain, fatigue, nausea, dyspnea, anxiety, depression, dementia, etc.).
2. Assist patient to achieve optimal level of comfort using a multidisciplinary approach.
3. Modify plan of care to achieve patient's optimal level of comfort (e.g., pharmacologic interventions, heat, cold, massage, positioning, touch, etc.).
4. Act as an advocate to help patient meet needs/goals, giving consideration to patient's rights.
5. Work on behalf of patient/family to identify and help resolve ethical and clinical concerns.
6. Provide a therapeutic environment, considering privacy, noise, light, visitors'/providers' patterns of interaction with patient, incorporation of pet therapy/music therapy, etc.
7. Recognize and incorporate diversity in the provision of patient care (e.g., ethnicity, gender, disability, spirituality, lifestyle, socioeconomic and education levels, etc.).
8. Support family involvement, in accordance with the patient's wishes, regarding caregiving and decision making.
9. Maintain an environment in which patient confidentiality is assured.
10. Acknowledge, respect, and support the emotional state of patient and/or family as they experience and/or express their emotions.
11. Identify need of patient/family for support systems/resources and make appropriate referrals.
12. Identify, acknowledge, support, and facilitate patient/family decisions regarding end-of-life care.

II. Teaching/Coaching Function

1. Assess the patient's and family's readiness and ability to learn.
2. Identify barriers to learning.
3. Encourage the patient's and family's participation in establishing educational goals.
4. Develop and implement an individualized teaching plan for patient and/or family.
5. Evaluate and modify teaching plan based on achievement of pre-established and ongoing learning needs.
6. Utilize opportunities for spontaneous education.
7. Teach patient and family about available community resources that they may need post-discharge.
8. Provide information and rationale related to diagnosis, procedures, self-care, prognosis, wellness, and modifiable risk factors.
9. Provide information in a sensitive manner to make culturally-avoided aspects of illness approachable and understandable.

III. Diagnostic and Patient Monitoring Function

1. Conduct and document a comprehensive assessment to obtain individual baseline data.
2. Reassess patient based on established standards and at appropriate intervals, using clinical judgment.
3. Use invasive and non-invasive methods to collect data.
4. Analyze all patient data in formulating a plan of care.
5. Develop an individualized plan of care.
6. Prioritize identified problems and modify the plan of care to achieve the best possible outcome.

7. Anticipate patient's responses and needs related to physiologic, psychosocial, spiritual, and cultural aspects of his/her illness.
8. Anticipate patient's response to treatment and monitor for potential problems.
9. Identify subtle changes in patient assessment to prevent deterioration of patient status.
10. Identify, document, and report deviations from expected findings.

IV. Administering and Monitoring Therapeutic Interventions

1. Administer medications using appropriate routes accurately and safely.
2. Monitor patient for therapeutic responses, reactions, untoward effects, toxicity, and incompatibilities of administered medications.
3. Maintain patent airway.
4. Take measures to ensure adequate oxygenation and gas exchange (e.g., suctioning, oxygen delivery, tracheostomy care, chest physical therapy, etc.).
5. Maintain effectiveness and patency of chest drainage systems.
6. Create and implement a wound management strategy that fosters healing, comfort, and appropriate drainage.
7. Monitor for signs and symptoms of infections and other complications.
8. Monitor and take measures to prevent alteration in skin integrity, including peristomal skin.
9. Maintain integrity and prevent infection of invasive drainage systems (e.g., catheters, percutaneous drains, etc.).
10. Appropriately and correctly use adaptive/assistive devices for mobility, immobility, positioning, and comfort.
11. Assess and monitor the effectiveness of adaptive/assistive devices.
12. Apply and/or monitor devices used to immobilize affected area (e.g., cast, splint, collar, etc.).
13. Perform neurovascular assessment of compromised extremity or other area.
14. Provide optimum nutrition during hospitalization, allowing for cultural and individual preferences.
15. Monitor effectiveness of nutritional interventions.
16. Initiate, maintain, and monitor intravenous therapy appropriately and correctly to minimize risks and prevent complications.
17. Maintain a safe environment.
18. Take measures to maintain adequate hydration and electrolyte balance.
19. Use existing guidelines/protocols/policies to respond to changing patient situations.

V. Effective Management of Rapidly Changing Situations

1. Coordinate complex situations by rapidly assessing priorities and delegating responsibilities to meet the needs of the patient and family.
2. Identify and manage a patient crisis.
3. Rapidly match demands and resources in emergency situations.
4. Initiate basic life support.
5. Use existing guidelines/protocols/policies to respond to urgent and emergent situations.

VI. Monitoring/Ensuring Quality Health Care Practices

1. Participate in quality improvement activities.
2. Collect and report data regarding system failures (e.g., safety, medication administration, chain of command, equipment, computer system, environment—loss of power, outlet failure, etc.).
3. Incorporate evidence-based practice into the patient's plan of care.
4. Question/clarify orders as appropriate.
5. Communicate clearly and concisely with health care team members to meet patient care needs.

VII. Organizational and Work-Role Competencies

1. Question/evaluate own practice based on established standards of care, review of the literature, research, and education.
2. Set priorities based on assignment, unit, and institutional needs.
3. Delegate patient care assignments based on competency levels and scope of practice of health care team members.
4. Follow institutional policies and procedures in response to an internal or external crisis or event.
5. Adhere to the *Scope and Standards of Medical-Surgical Nursing Practice*.
6. Practice in accordance with the rules and regulations of state board of nursing in state(s) of licensure.
7. Use the chain of command appropriately in own work setting.
8. Recognize unsafe work practices (e.g., nurse/patient ratio, ergonomics, standard precautions, etc.) and appropriately intervene.
9. Incorporate strategies that support effective team dynamics in a caring and nurturing environment.
10. Participate in health-related community activities (e.g., health fairs, voting, and walks).

Adapted from Benner, P. (1984). *From novice to expert: Excellence and power in clinical nursing practice.* Menlo Park, CA: Addison-Wesley.

The following are individual questions.

1. The nurse recognizes the patient **most likely** to experience hypercarbic respiratory failure is the one with a diagnosis of:
   a. acute respiratory distress syndrome.
   b. pulmonary embolus.
   c. bronchitis.
   d. pulmonary edema.

2. A patient with Stage II adenocarcinoma of the lung is being treated with the anti-tumor antibiotic doxorubicin (Adriamycin®). The nurse knows that alteration in dose scheduling of doxorubicin is needed to decrease the risk for toxicity to which of the following organs?
   a. Liver
   b. Heart
   c. Pancreas
   d. Kidney

3. A 57-year-old patient is admitted to the medical unit for progressive symptoms of dyspnea on exertion and decreased appetite, and is scheduled for pulmonary function testing. When the patient asks what the test will measure, the nurse's response is based on the knowledge that the tests are used to identify which three general patterns of pulmonary abnormality?
   a. Obstructive, restrictive, and mixed
   b. Obstructive, constrictive, and mixed
   c. Restrictive, functional, and mixed
   d. Constrictive, functional, and mixed

4. The preferred Mantoux test for screening and diagnosis of tuberculosis should be read by the trained nurse in:
   a. 18 to 24 hours.
   b. 24 to 36 hours.
   c. 48 to 72 hours.
   d. 72 to 96 hours.

5. Arterial blood gas results, including a pH less than 7.35 and a pCO_2 greater than 45, would reflect:
   a. metabolic acidosis.
   b. respiratory acidosis.
   c. metabolic alkalosis.
   d. respiratory alkalosis.

6. For the patient with a new tracheostomy, the nurse must be alert to which **early** complication?
   a. Decannulation
   b. Infection
   c. Bleeding
   d. Tracheomalacia

7. A 32-year-old patient on the medical unit experiences an acute asthma episode. All of the following are ordered to treat the patient. What will the nurse administer **first**?
   a. Intravenous corticosteroids
   b. Oxygen by nasal cannula
   c. Bronchodilator by metered-dose inhaler
   d. Intravenous fluids

8. In discussing long-term disease management with a 23-year-old patient with cystic fibrosis (CF), the nurse provides dietary instruction to decrease the risk of which common complication of CF associated with mineral malabsorption?
   a. Hyperlipidemia
   b. Neutropenia
   c. Thrombocytopenia
   d. Osteopenia

9. The nurse discusses the potential side effects of etoposide (Etopophos®) with a patient diagnosed with small cell carcinoma of the lung. Which of the following should be identified?
   a. Diarrhea
   b. Hypotension
   c. Nasal congestion
   d. Dry cough

The next two questions pertain to the following scenario.

William Mathis, age 55, has been receiving external radiation to the chest following surgery for non-small cell cancer of the lung. He presents for radiation one morning and reports a sore throat. His oral mucosa is swollen and red with ulcerations, and his saliva is thick and ropy.

10. What intervention does the nurse teach Mr. Mathis?
    a. Rinse his mouth before and after meals and at bedtime with a solution of salt and sodium bicarbonate.
    b. Gargle and rinse his mouth four times daily with a commercial antiseptic mouthwash.
    c. Maintain a diet of warm, bland liquids until the ulcerations heal.
    d. Use a soft-bristled toothbrush dipped in hydrogen peroxide to clean his teeth and tongue.

11. Mr. Mathis tells the nurse that he is so tired he can hardly get up in the morning. Which of the following interventions is an appropriate goal for Mr. Mathis?
    a. Eliminate all unnecessary activity until radiation is completed.
    b. Establish a daily walking program.
    c. Consult with a psychiatrist regarding situational depression.
    d. Begin rigorous aerobic exercise several times a week.

The next three questions pertain to the following scenario.

Mr. Gordon Bruce, age 82, is admitted to the medical unit with a diagnosis of pneumonia.

12. The nurse knows that Mr. Bruce's risk of developing pneumonia was increased because admission assessment revealed he also:
    a. is homebound.
    b. has diabetes mellitus.
    c. is African-American.
    d. has a Stage II decubitus ulcer.

13. Mr. Bruce develops a large pleural effusion that affects his respiratory function. The physician performs a thoracentesis in the patient's room. Which post-procedure symptom would the nurse report immediately to the physician?
    a. Patient complaint of productive cough
    b. Respiratory rate of 16 breaths per minute
    c. Patient complaint of chest tightness
    d. Heart rate of 72 beats per minute

14. After Mr. Bruce is afebrile for 24 hours, the attending physician recommends that the patient receive the pneumococcal vaccine (Pneumovax®). In accordance with administration guidelines, the nurse would deliver the vaccine by:
    a. subcutaneous injection into the patient's abdomen.
    b. intramuscular injection into the patient's mid-lateral thigh.
    c. intravenous injection into the patient's antecubital space.
    d. intradermal injection into the patient's forearm.

The following are individual questions.

15. To confirm a patient's diagnosis of pulmonary tuberculosis, the nurse will be asked to collect a sputum specimen for:
    a. culture and sensitivity.
    b. *Pneumocystis carinii.*
    c. acid-fast bacillus.
    d. *Haemophilus influenzae.*

16. A patient is scheduled to undergo bronchoscopy. The nurse will anticipate an order to hold which of the following medications on the morning of the procedure?
    a. Ibuprofen (Motrin®)
    b. Atenolol (Tenormin®)
    c. Omeprazole (Prilosec®)
    d. Digoxin (Lanoxin®)

17. In following guidelines from the Centers for Disease Control and Prevention (CDC) on the medical unit, the nurse knows that the patient with pulmonary tuberculosis must be placed on which type of precaution?
    a. Droplet
    b. Contact
    c. Airborne
    d. Reverse

18. A patient is being monitored via continuous pulse oximetry. The nurse knows that pulse oximetry results are most likely to be affected by the patient's:
    a. heart rate.
    b. gender.
    c. blood glucose.
    d. skin pigmentation.

19. A patient is admitted to the medical unit with a Heimlich valve. The nurse recognizes this as an intervention used for:
    a. administration of chemotherapeutic agents.
    b. uncomplicated hemothorax.
    c. post-herpetic neuralgia.
    d. administration of intrapleural antibiotics.

20. Nursing care of the patient who has had a bronchoscopy includes keeping the patient:
    a. NPO until the gag reflex returns.
    b. in the dorsal recumbent position until fully recovered from sedation.
    c. free of secretions by using an oral suction device.
    d. in a lateral position to keep the dressing dry and intact.

21. The drug of choice for treating latent tuberculosis (TB) infection, such as found in associates of a person newly diagnosed with tuberculosis, is:
    a. kanamycin (Kantrex®).
    b. isoniazid (INH®).
    c. cycloserine (Seromycin®).
    d. streptomycin sulfate.

22. Fluctuations or tidaling may be seen in the water seal chamber of a patient with a chest tube because:
    a. there is a kink in the tubing.
    b. the patient's lungs have re-expanded.
    c. suction is being used.
    d. respirations cause pressure changes in the patient's pleural space.

23. The nurse identifies which of the following individuals as at greatest risk to develop pneumonia?
    a. 25-year-old who has recently given birth
    b. 35-year-old who is recovering from a laparoscopic cholecystectomy
    c. 55-year-old who recently fractured a fibula
    d. 65-year-old who has the flu

24. Montelukast (Singulair®) or another leukotriene modifier may be prescribed for the patient with asthma to:
    a. inhibit a nonproductive cough.
    b. reverse bronchospasm during an acute attack.
    c. prevent bronchoconstriction and inflammation.
    d. decrease viscosity of mucous.

25. In teaching a patient about the use of the Advair Diskus®, the nurse should include which of the following instructions?
    a. Take two puffs at the first sign of an asthma attack.
    b. Rinse your mouth after using the inhaler.
    c. The inhaler can be used for only 3 months after removal from the foil wrapper.
    d. More frequent dosing may be required if you have diabetes.

26. A patient with squamous cell carcinoma of the lung is readmitted to the hospital midway through her third cycle of chemotherapy with a diagnosis of neutropenia. Vital signs include temperature 100.6 degrees F; pulse 84 beats per minute, regular; respirations 24 breaths per minute. The most appropriate interpretation of these findings is that:
    a. the patient may have an upper respiratory infection.
    b. the patient is having a normal reaction to cancer that often increases the patient's metabolic rate.
    c. systemic chemotherapy often causes a slight increase in vital signs.
    d. further assessment is needed immediately because a medical emergency may be occurring.

27. Bronchoconstriction with hyperresponsiveness of the airways in the patient with asthma is characterized by which of the following?
    a. PEFR of 100 to 150 L/minute
    b. SaO_2 of 88%
    c. Interstitial infiltrates on chest X-ray
    d. FEV1 of 80% predicted

28. When a pulse oximetry monitor indicates that a patient has a drop in SpO_2 from 96% to 85% over 4 hours, the nurse will **first**:
    a. request an order for stat arterial blood gases.
    b. start the patient on oxygen by nasal cannula at 2 L/minute.
    c. notify the physician of the change.
    d. check the position of the probe on the patient's finger or earlobe.

29. In teaching a patient how to use cromolyn (Intal®) when exercising, the nurse instructs him to:
    a. omit the usual dose of medication if planning to exercise within 1 hour.
    b. double the dose of medication on the morning when exercise is planned.
    c. wait until after exercising to take the medication.
    d. take the medication 10 to 20 minutes before exercising.

30. Data that contribute to the diagnosis of chronic bronchitis include:
    a. documentation of blebs and bullae on chest X-ray.
    b. report of chronic productive cough from December through February in the past two winters.
    c. elevation of arterial CO_2 for more than one month.
    d. evidence of hyperinflated alveoli on chest X-ray.

31. An individual with an onset of emphysema before age 40 should be assessed for:
    a. alpha-antitrypsin deficiency.
    b. cystic fibrosis.
    c. diabetes mellitus.
    d. Tay Sachs disease.

32. An advantage of using positive end-expiratory pressure (PEEP) for a patient who is being mechanically ventilated is that PEEP:
    a. decreases the risk of barotraumas.
    b. increases cardiac output.
    c. promotes gas exchange by preventing alveolar collapse.
    d. is effective for the patient with compliant lungs.

33. The nurse caring for the patient who is being mechanically ventilated becomes concerned about the endotracheal (ET) tube position when the patient's:
    a. respiratory rate increases above baseline.
    b. breaths are not synchronous with the ventilator.
    c. need for suctioning increases.
    d. chest movement is uneven.

34. An adult patient will be placed on droplet precautions if diagnosed with which of the following?
    a. Meningococal pneumonia
    b. Pneumococcal pneumonia
    c. Respiratory syncytial virus (RSV)
    d. Varicella zoster

35. A patient is to have a ventilation/perfusion (V/Q) scan. The nurse knows this study has been ordered to diagnose:
    a. asthma.
    b. pulmonary fibrosis.
    c. pulmonary embolus.
    d. COPD.

36. Arterial blood gas results that are characteristic of late-stage COPD include which of the following?
    a. pH 7.25, $PaCO_2$ 60 mm Hg, PaO_2 60 mm Hg, HCO_3 30 mEq/L
    b. pH 7.30, $PaCO_2$ 45 mm Hg, PaO_2 60 mm Hg, HCO_3 18 mEq/L
    c. pH 7.45, $PaCO_2$ 40 mm Hg, PaO_2 75 mm Hg, HCO_3 26 mEq/L
    d. pH 7.50, $PaCO_2$ 30 mm Hg, PaO_2 80 mm Hg, HCO_3 35 mEq/L

37. A technique the nurse should teach a patient with COPD to promote expiration is:
    a. diaphragmatic breathing.
    b. to exhale quickly.
    c. pursed-lip breathing.
    d. to inhale quickly and deeply.

38. In monitoring the use of a non-rebreather mask for the delivery of oxygen, the nurse knows that it:
    a. provides 40% to 60% oxygen concentration.
    b. is used to give oxygen quickly.
    c. is the most comfortable for the patient to use.
    d. provides the highest concentration of oxygen.

39. On assessment, the nurse determines that a patient has marked dyspnea and impending respiratory failure. Findings include which of the following?
    a. Bilateral inspiratory and expiratory wheezing
    b. Significantly decreased breath sounds with no wheezing
    c. Diaphragmatic breathing
    d. Respiratory rate of 30 breaths per minute

40. When preparing a patient for a pulmonary angiogram, the nurse:
    a. assesses the patient for iodine allergy.
    b. informs the patient that he will be NPO after midnight.
    c. obtains an informed consent.
    d. withholds all patient medications until after the procedure.

41. The best approach to patient teaching when a patient has a pulmonary disease is to:
    a. use a family member to translate information if the patient does not speak English.
    b. inform the patient to go to the Emergency Department if he does not understand the instructions after arriving home.
    c. assess the patient's need before developing an education plan.
    d. use print media with pictures as the best source of information.

42. A patient tells the nurse that he thinks he has sleep apnea because his wife complains about his snoring. The nurse knows that sleep apnea also is suggested by the patient's history of:
    a. sleeping on a hard mattress.
    b. frequent awakenings at night.
    c. asthma.
    d. cough.

43. Arterial blood gas results seen early in an acute asthma attack include:
    a. pH 7.25, $PaCO_2$ 60 mm Hg, PaO_2 60 mm Hg.
    b. pH 7.35, $PaCO_2$ 45 mm Hg, PaO_2 75 mm Hg.
    c. pH 7.48, $PaCO_2$ 30 mm Hg, PAO_2 75 mm Hg.
    d. PH 7.50, $PaCO_2$ 30 mm Hg, PaO_2 80 mm Hg.

44. When teaching the patient with asthma about the use of the peak flow meter, the nurse instructs the patient to:
    a. increase the use of quick-relief medications if the meter indicates the yellow zone.
    b. carry the flow meter at all times.
    c. close the mouth around the mouthpiece and inhale quickly when using the flow meter.
    d. go the emergency room if the meter indicates the yellow zone.

45. To decrease a patient's shortness of breath and a sense of impending doom during an asthma attack, the nurse will:
    a. place the patient on a cardiac monitor and observe from the nurses' station.
    b. let the patient rest alone in a quiet, calm environment.
    c. reassure the patient that the doctor will arrive soon.
    d. stay with the patient and encourage pursed-lip breathing.

46. In providing patient education about influenza, the nurse identifies which of the following as a potential contraindication to vaccination?
    a. Severe allergy to milk or milk products
    b. Household contact with someone 50 years of age or older
    c. Past reaction to pneumococcal vaccine
    d. Development of Guillain-Barré syndrome within 6 weeks of previous vaccination

47. To help a patient stop smoking, the nurse tells the patient that the most successful programs for smoking cessation include:
    a. self-help programs and support groups.
    b. psychotherapy.
    c. hypnosis.
    d. behavior modification and nicotine replacement.

48. The nutritional needs of a patient with chronic obstructive pulmonary disease (COPD) include:
    a. a high-carbohydrate, low-fat diet.
    b. a high-protein, low-fat diet.
    c. eating cold foods rather than hot foods.
    d. eating foods that require less chewing.

49. When the patient asks what causes the lung destruction of emphysema, the nurse tells the patient it is a result of:
    a. air trapping in distal alveoli.
    b. decreased vital capacity.
    c. constriction of small bronchioles.
    d. decreased tidal volume.

50. A patient complains of a knife-like chest pain of sudden onset. The nurse suspects that this is **most likely** due to:
    a. acute respiratory distress syndrome.
    b. exacerbation of emphysema.
    c. worsening hypoxia with pneumonia.
    d. pulmonary embolus.

Cardiovascular   Questions 51-85

The next three questions pertain to the following scenario.

Matthew Bourne, age 65, has been diagnosed with stage 2 primary hypertension. Mr. Bourne is to begin taking a thiazide diuretic and labetolol (Normodyne®), a beta-adrenergic antagonist.

51. Which instruction should the nurse emphasize when teaching Mr. Bourne about labetolol?
    a. Take the medication between meals.
    b. Drink at least 3 liters of fluid daily.
    c. Have your vision checked regularly.
    d. Change positions very slowly.

52. Which of the following puts Mr. Bourne at risk for primary hypertension?
    a. Body mass index of 24
    b. One beer daily
    c. Walks for 30 minutes daily
    d. Eats fast food twice a week

Mr. Bourne later reports that he has stopped taking the labetolol because it interfered with his social life.

53. Which response by the nurse is most appropriate in response to Mr. Bourne's statement?
    a. "Many men stop taking their blood pressure medications due to changes in sexual functioning. Have you had this problem?"
    b. "Often these drugs cause fatigue, but the dosage can be adjusted to correct this side effect."
    c. "What exactly do you mean by social life?"
    d. "Never stop taking blood pressure medication suddenly because this can be dangerous."

The next three questions pertain to the following scenario.

Janice Elliot, age 72, has been admitted to the hospital with a diagnosis of unstable angina. She is receiving oxygen at 3 liters per minute by nasal cannula and has a saline lock in place. Telemetry monitoring shows she is in sinus tachycardia with a rate of 112 beats per minute. Ms. Elliot also has sublingual nitroglycerin at the bedside for use as needed.

54. Based on this patient's diagnosis, the nurse caring for Mrs. Elliot recognizes that she:
    a. only experiences chest pain with strenuous activity.
    b. has unpredictable frequency or intensity of symptoms.
    c. will have pathologic Q-waves on her cardiac rhythm strip.
    d. has altered contractility of her ventricles.

55. Mrs. Elliot's rapid heart rate may be a problem primarily because it:
    a. places her at risk for pulmonary emboli.
    b. can cause extreme shortness of breath.
    c. can result in altered cardiac output.
    d. further narrows her coronary arteries.

56. The nurse teaches Mrs. Elliot about nitroglycerin. Following the teaching session, it is **most important** for the patient to:
    a. indicate that she will call for help if three nitroglycerin tablets don't relieve her chest pain.
    b. verbalize that flushing and dizziness are common side effects of the drug.

c. verbalize understanding that nitroglycerin will help prevent her from having a myocardial infarction (MI).

d. indicate that she will not take the drug unless she is experiencing chest pain.

The next four questions pertain to the following scenario.

Geneva Curry, age 65, is transferred to a medical telemetry unit after several days in the coronary care unit for treatment of an acute MI. Ms. Curry remains very anxious, with occasional episodes of chest pressure.

57. Which medication does the nurse prepare for Ms. Curry to decrease her anxiety and improve cardiac output?
    a. Nitroprusside (Nipride®)
    b. Diazepam (Valium®)
    c. Morphine sulfate (MS)
    d. Dopamine (Intropin®)

58. The nurse closely monitors Ms. Curry for which common complication of MI?
    a. Cardiogenic shock
    b. Dysrhythmias
    c. Valvular rupture
    d. Cardiac tamponade

59. Ms. Curry's temperature rises to 100.4 degrees F. The nurse interprets this finding as:
    a. evidence of pericarditis.
    b. evidence of infection.
    c. due to myocardial injury.
    d. due to probable dehydration.

60. Which of the following activities will the nurse plan for Ms. Curry as part of her rehabilitation?
    a. Bedrest for 24 hours after transfer
    b. Bathroom privileges and self-care activities
    c. Unsupervised ambulation for distances less than 200 feet
    d. Ad lib activities with cardiac telemetry monitoring

The next four questions pertain to the following scenario.

Fernando Rivera, age 50, is admitted with complaints of severe pressure in his chest and shortness of breath. Mr. Rivera is stabilized and scheduled for a cardiac catheterization with possible percutaneous transluminal coronary angioplasty (PTCA).

61. During the pre-procedure instructions, Mr. Rivera asks the nurse to review the reasons for the cardiac catheterization. The nurse's response is based on an understanding that this procedure is performed to:
    a. determine if any blockages are present in the coronary arteries and test for sensitivity to thrombolytic agents.
    b. measure the amount of blood being pumped from his heart.

c. determine if any structural defects are present in his heart.
d. visualize any blockages in the coronary arteries and dilate any obstructed arteries with a small balloon.

62. Which of the following is the **most critical** assessment that the nurse should make prior to Mr. Rivera's cardiac catheterization?
    a. Peripheral pulse rates
    b. Height and weight
    c. Allergy to iodine or shellfish
    d. Intake and output

Mr. Rivera's recovery following PTCA is uncomplicated.

63. The nurse instructs Mr. Rivera regarding risk factor modification to prevent stenosis. Which of the following is most important in prevention of re-stenosis?
    a. Abstinence from alcohol
    b. 1 hour of daily aerobic exercise
    c. Stress management
    d. Smoking cessation

64. At discharge, the nurse instructs Mr. Rivera about the use of nitroglycerin. Following instruction, it is **most important** that the patient verbalize:
    a. the need to seek medical attention if chest pain or discomfort is not relieved by three nitroglycerin tablets.
    b. the possible adverse effects of nitroglycerin.
    c. the need for lifelong use of nitroglycerin to prevent a heart attack.
    d. that he is to use nitroglycerin only if chest pain occurs.

The next five questions pertain to the following scenario.

Herbert Chang, age 64, has been diagnosed with congestive heart failure as a result of a recent anterior wall myocardial infarction. He is being transferred from the critical care area to the medical-surgical unit. Current medications include lisinopril (Prinivil®) 20 mg by mouth twice daily; digoxin (Lanoxin®) 0.125 mg by mouth daily; furosemide (Lasix®) 40 mg by mouth daily; potassium chloride (K-Dur®) 20 mEq by mouth twice daily.

65. The nurse will instruct Mr. Chang to immediately report which symptom?
    a. Frequent urination
    b. Shortness of breath
    c. Diarrhea
    d. Nausea

66. Which nursing intervention is **most important** to Mr. Chang's improved condition?
    a. Monitoring fluid intake and output
    b. Limiting the number of family visits
    c. Assessing the patient's knowledge of the disease
    d. Encouraging coughing and deep breathing

67. The nurse's assessment of Mr. Chang's response to digoxin will include which of the following as the **most common** early indicator of toxicity?
    a. Diarrhea and abdominal discomfort
    b. Anorexia
    c. Headache
    d. Visual disturbance and confusion

68. The nurse also is aware that some medications can increase serum digitalis concentrations. These include:
    a. rifampicin (Rifadin®) and neomycin (Neomix®).
    b. cholestyramine (Questran®) and colestipol (Colestid®).
    c. sulfasalazine (Azulfidine®) and metoclopramide (Reglan®).
    d. amiodarone (Cordarone®) and diltiazem (Cardizem®).

69. In preparing Mr. Chang for discharge, the nurse will reinforce the importance of which of the following?
    a. Fluid restriction
    b. Activity limitations
    c. Daily weights
    d. Carbohydrate elimination

The following are individual items.

70. A 68-year-old female is admitted with a diagnosis of congestive heart failure and ischemic cardiomyopathy. Her cardiac history includes three previous myocardial infarctions and three coronary artery bypass grafts. The patient is still able to eat. Which dietary restriction would best apply for this patient?
    a. Low cholesterol
    b. Restricted sodium
    c. Low fat
    d. Reduced calorie

71. A 65-year-old male is diagnosed with right-sided heart failure and admitted to the medical-surgical unit. Based on this diagnosis, the nurse will expect assessment to include which of the following findings?
    a. Dyspnea on exertion and bibasilar crackles
    b. Distended veins and systolic murmur
    c. Dependent edema and hepatic engorgement
    d. Cool extremities and weak peripheral pulses

72. A patient is admitted to the hospital after experiencing substernal chest pain for 2 hours. Which laboratory study does the nurse recognize as **most useful** in determining whether the patient has experienced a myocardial infarction?
    a. Complete blood count (CBC) with differential
    b. C-reactive protein (CRP)
    c. Troponin
    d. Homocysteine

73. The priority nursing care for a patient with suspected myocardial infarction is:
    a. auscultating for adventitious breath sounds.
    b. monitoring fluid and electrolyte status.
    c. preventing thrombi and emboli.
    d. providing appropriate analgesia.

74. Minimally invasive direct coronary artery bypass grafting (MIDCABG) may be recommended for the patient who meets which of the following criteria?
    a. Single vessel coronary artery disease
    b. Age less than 40 years
    c. Excessive risk for traditional CABG
    d. Presence of both valvular and coronary artery disease

75. The nurse recognizes the most common clinical finding of left-sided heart failure as:
    a. S3 gallop.
    b. sinus bradycardia.
    c. fever.
    d. ascites.

76. The nurse should teach the patient with a permanent pacemaker for treatment of sinus node dysfunction how to:
    a. change the batteries.
    b. monitor the pulse.
    c. change setting from demand to continuous.
    d. strengthen the sinoatrial (SA) node.

The next two questions pertain to the following scenario.

Stephanie Pompey, age 45, is diagnosed with primary hypertension. Ms. Pompey is prescribed a combination treatment for hypertension that includes furosemide (Lasix®) 40 mg daily and captopril (Capoten®) 20 mg three times daily.

77. Which of the following must be specifically assessed to determine if complications of hypertension are imminent?
    a. Dizziness
    b. Tinnitus
    c. Chest pain
    d. Leg cramps

78. Nursing instruction on medication management for Ms. Pompey includes which of the following?
    a. Captopril is best administered immediately after meals.
    b. Antihypertensive medications should not be discontinued without the physician's permission.
    c. Captopril is best absorbed if taken with orange juice.
    d. Dosage of antihypertensive medications can be adjusted based on home BP readings.

The next two questions pertain to the following scenario.

Edward Pelletier, age 65, has been recently prescribed telmisartan (Micardis HCT®) for treatment of primary hypertension.

79. What should the nurse emphasize in teaching Mr. Pelletier about his new medication?
    a. Take the medication twice daily before meals.
    b. Inform your doctor if you are also taking a diuretic.
    c. Continue to take your lithium as prescribed.
    d. Avoid acetaminophen (Tylenol®) usage while taking telmisartan.

80. The nurse's discussion of the drug's action with Mr. Pelletier is based on knowledge that telmisartan is a/an:
    a. beta adrenergic blocker.
    b. calcium channel blocker.
    c. angiotensin II receptor blocker.
    d. angiotensin converting enzyme inhibitor.

The following are individual items.

81. The nurse expects to administer which of the following drugs to a patient with dilated cardiomyopathy?
    a. Adenosine (Adenocard®)
    b. Nitroglycerine (Nitro-Bid®)
    c. Procainamide (Pronestyl®)
    d. Digoxin (Lanoxin®)

82. The nurse understands the reason for administering enalapril (Vasotec®) to a patient with dilated cardiomyopathy as:
    a. preventing thrombus formation.
    b. preventing dysrhythmias.
    c. reducing peripheral blood pressure.
    d. reducing heart rate.

83. The nurse correctly recognizes the **most effective** treatment for ventricular fibrillation as:
    a. amiodarone (Cordarone®).
    b. atenolol (Tenormin®).
    c. defibrillation.
    d. cardiac catheterization.

84. Following an acute myocardial infarction (AMI), a 68-year-old patient is being prepared for hospital discharge. In accordance with standards of care for the patient with AMI, the nurse knows that discharge orders may include which of the following medications?
    a. Nifedipine (Procardia®)
    b. Amiodarone (Cordarone®)
    c. Verapamil (Calan®)
    d. Carvedilol (Coreg®)

85. The nurse recognizes that a patient is at risk to develop infective endocarditis if he has which of the following conditions?
    a. Diabetes mellitus
    b. Acquired valvular disease
    c. Cardiomyopathy
    d. Myocardial infarction

The following are individual questions.

86. The nurse recognizes which of the following as goals for treatment of the patient with acute pancreatitis?
    a. Manage pain and increase pancreatic secretions.
    b. Hydrate aggressively to decrease serum calcium levels.
    c. Increase fluid volume and decrease pancreatic enzymes.
    d. Administer steroids to decrease pancreatic inflammation.

87. A patient on the medical unit has been diagnosed with *Clostridium difficile* colitis. What abnormalities would the nurse expect to see in the patient's laboratory results?
    a. Decreased platelet count
    b. Leukocytosis
    c. Decreased serum creatinine
    d. Hyperalbuminemia

88. A 29-year-old female is admitted to the medical unit with diagnosis of abdominal pain. Admitting vital signs include temperature 101.4 degrees F; pulse 118 beats per minute; respirations 26 breaths per minute; blood pressure 78/46 mm Hg with a mean arterial pressure (MAP) of 52. With this MAP value, the nurse recognizes the patient is at risk for:
    a. dehydration.
    b. multi-organ failure.
    c. metabolic alkalosis.
    d. ileus.

89. A 38-year-old patient with hepatitis B asks the nurse how he could have contracted the disease. The nurse's response is based on knowledge that the causative virus is transmitted:
    a. orally through fecal contamination.
    b. through improper food handling.
    c. through sexual contact.
    d. by eating raw shellfish.

90. In the patient with liver disease, the nurse knows that which of the following is suggestive of portal hypertension?
    a. Ascites and tarry stools
    b. Ascites and malodorous urine
    c. Increased white blood cell count
    d. Increased platelet count

91. A 52-year-old patient with chronic liver disease exhibits early common signs of hepatic encephalopathy, including which of the following?
    a. Aphagia
    b. Personality changes
    c. Seizures
    d. Rancid breath odor

92. Nursing interventions and orders for a patient following a barium swallow should include which of the following?
    a. Decreased fluids and increased activity
    b. Increased fluids and decreased activity
    c. Increased fluids and a laxative
    d. Decreased fluids and a laxative

93. The nurse has admitted a male patient with recurrent epigastric pain. He complains of substernal burning, belching, and regurgitation of undigested food when lying down. The nurse suspects these complaints most likely indicate:
    a. duodenal ulcer.
    b. gastric cancer.
    c. peptic ulcer disease.
    d. gastroesophageal reflux disease.

94. A patient with dyspepsia asks about herbal products or dietary supplements that may decrease symptoms. The nurse suggests the patient speak with the health care provider about use of:
    a. caraway oil.
    b. fish oil.
    c. saw palmetto.
    d. black cohosh.

95. The nurse is teaching the patient and family about managing peptic ulcer disease. It is important to include which of the following as part of the dietary instruction?
    a. Have a bedtime snack regularly.
    b. Take caffeine-containing beverages in moderation.
    c. Eat very large meals to alleviate disease symptoms.
    d. Eat quickly to prevent overdistention and reflux.

96. The **most sensitive** indicator of blood loss during an acute GI bleed is:
    a. metabolic acidosis.
    b. oxygen saturation.
    c. hemoglobin and hematocrit.
    d. vasomotor instability.

97. A patient has a nasogatric tube to low constant suction following a partial gastrectomy with a vagotomy. Following standards of practice, the nurse would question the surgeon about which of the following postoperative orders?
    a. Notify physician for a temperature over 101.5 degrees F.
    b. Call physician for any bright red blood from the nasogastric tube.
    c. Irrigate the nasogastric tube with 30 ml of normal saline every shift.
    d. Keep the nasogastric tube taped and secured to the patient's nares.

The next three questions pertain to the following scenario.

Mr. Theodore Lawson, age 45, is seen preoperatively for placement of a colostomy.

98. The nurse recognizes that an important factor in determining site placement for an ostomy is:
    a. patient gender.
    b. presence of skin folds.
    c. surgeon preference.
    d. stage of disease process.

99. Mr. Lawson expresses concern about his sexual functioning following the ostomy placement. The nurse tells him that:
    a. male impotence is not common.
    b. sexual function is reduced.
    c. his surgeon can discuss effects of the procedure.
    d. libido will not be affected.

100. Mr. Lawson also asks about irritation related to stool contact with peristomal skin. The nurse explains that:
    a. peristomal skin will adapt to stool contact and no adjustments are needed.
    b. worrying increases ostomy drainage and should be avoided if the skin is to heal.
    c. proper sizing of the ostomy wafer is important to prevent stool contact with the skin.
    d. peristomal irritation is unusual and would require stoma revision.

The next five questions pertain to the following scenario.

Ms. Becky Gresham, age 24, had ileostomy placement 2 days ago.

101. The nursing assistant reports Ms. Gresham's output over 24 hours to be 2,000 cc and informs the nurse that the patient is experiencing nausea and vomiting. The nurse knows that this:
    a. is rare after surgery but can be treated with antiemetics.
    b. can place Ms. Gresham at risk for dehydration.
    c. is a sign of ileostomy rejection.
    d. can increase the likelihood that Ms. Gresham will develop constipation.

102. When administering medications to Ms. Gresham, the nurse knows that:
    a. no modifications are required because the distal colon remains intact.
    b. oral medications are safe as long as they are enteric-coated.
    c. medications must be administered on an empty stomach to maximize absorption.
    d. liquid or chewable forms are preferred for Ms. Gresham.

103. The nurse who teaches Ms. Gresham about ileostomy drainage will ensure that the patient understands:
    a. ileostomy drainage has a strong, foul-smelling odor.
    b. the drainage eventually will attain the consistency of soft stool.
    c. drainage will remain somewhat liquefied.
    d. the drainage has no odor if the bag is emptied frequently.

104. Ms. Gresham asks if she will need to modify her diet due to the ileostomy. The nurse tells her that she should:
    a. eat slowly and chew food thoroughly.
    b. include high fiber early to promote bowel activity.
    c. require no restrictions once her surgical site is healed.
    d. restrict fluids to reduce watery output.

105. The nurse teaches Ms. Gresham to care for her ileostomy by:
    a. irrigating the stoma daily until continence is established.
    b. changing the pouch daily.
    c. using skin barrier only when irritation develops.
    d. changing ostomy pouch when the stoma is inactive.

The next three questions pertain to the following scenario.

Ms. Jeanne Boland, age 20, is admitted to the hospital with symptoms of inflammatory bowel disease (IBD). She will undergo testing to determine if her symptoms are suggestive of Crohn's disease or ulcerative colitis.

106. In response to Ms. Boland's questions, the nurse confirms that testing for IBD is **unlikely** to include:
    a. routine colonoscopy.
    b. barium enema.
    c. stool exam and culture.
    d. serum albumin.

107. In discussing Crohn's disease, the nurse tells Ms. Boland that:
    a. a high-fat diet often is linked to its onset.
    b. pain is commonly on the left side.
    c. intestinal strictures commonly result.
    d. methotrexate often is prescribed for bowel inflammation.

108. The nurse knows that treatment for Crohn's disease may include which of the following?
    a. Elimination of all fatty foods
    b. Bowel rest and elemental diet
    c. High-fiber diet
    d. Low-protein diet

The following are individual items.

109. A 54-year-old with suspected gastrointestinal (GI) bleeding undergoes diagnostic endoscopy, which determines that the site of bleeding is a duodenal ulcer. The nurse explains to the patient that most bleeding ulcers are related to the patient's:
    a. intake of spicy foods.
    b. use of salicylates.
    c. history of smoking.
    d. severe retching and vomiting.

110. When the patient with acute pancreatitis complains of abdominal pain, the nurse can suggest which position to best decrease tension on the abdomen?
    a. Side-lying with head elevated 45 degrees
    b. Supine with knees extended
    c. Prone decubitus
    d. Modified trendelenberg

The next three questions pertain to the following scenario.

Marcus Ripley, age 56, was admitted to the medical unit after 2 days of nausea, vomiting, and diarrhea at home. Small bowel obstruction is suspected. A nasogastric tube is inserted to suction, and a liter of lactated ringers is hung. The patient is allowed nothing by mouth (NPO), and antiemetic medications are ordered.

111. The nurse will monitor Mr. Ripley for potential complications of the nasogastric tube, including:
    a. gastrocolic reflux.
    b. sinusitis.
    c. esophageal erosion.
    d. aspiration.

112. Laboratory staff call to report the result of Mr. Ripley's recent blood work as potassium 2.8 mEq/liter. The nurse recognizes the patient's hypokalemia as most likely due to the:
    a. type and rate of intravenous fluid.
    b. patient's inability to take anything by mouth.
    c. type and sequence of blood draws.
    d. patient's vomiting and nasogastric output.

113. The diagnosis of small bowel obstruction due to adhesions is confirmed by CT scan. Mr. Ripley recovers after 3 days of bowel rest without surgical intervention. To limit potential reoccurrence, the nurse's discharge instructions for diet will identify the patient's need to maintain a:
    a. high-fiber diet.
    b. low-fat diet.
    c. low-residue diet.
    d. high-potassium diet.

The next six questions pertain to the following scenario.

Charlotte Simpson, age 62, is admitted to the surgical unit after a gastric resection for gastric cancer.

114. Ms. Simpson has a nasogastric tube in place with minimal output. When she complains of nausea, the nurse administers an antiemetic as ordered. However, the patient's nausea continues. The nurse should:
    a. flush the tube with 30 cc of normal saline.
    b. reposition the tube 1 inch further into the patient's stomach fundus.
    c. flush the tube with 30 cc of dextrose solution.
    d. reposition the tube 1 inch away from the patient's stomach wall.

115. Ms. Simpson states that she doesn't want anyone to see her in this condition, even her husband. The nurse's **best** response is:
    a. "Patients' rights protect your privacy. I won't allow anyone in."
    b. "I've seen gastric cancer patients who look much worse. Don't worry."
    c. "Would you like to talk to a social worker?"
    d. "What about your condition worries you?"

116. On the second postoperative day, Ms. Simpson's urinary output is 50 cc/hour. Her heart rate is 134 beats per minute, and her blood pressure is 90/56 mm Hg. The nurse recognizes these findings as consistent with:
    a. gastric outlet syndrome.
    b. third spacing.
    c. vagal rebound.
    d. pyloric stimulation.

117. Ms. Simpson improves, and the nurse prepares her for hospital discharge on the sixth postoperative day. Which point about dumping syndrome should the nurse include in discharge teaching?
    a. Eat a 10-gram low-fat diet.
    b. Drink 8 ounces of water with each meal.
    c. Eat six small meals per day.
    d. Make high-carbohydrate food selections.

One year later, Ms. Simpson is readmitted to the surgical unit with recurrent gastric cancer and gastric outlet obstruction. A percutaneous endoscopic gastrostomy (PEG) tube and a jejunostomy tube (J-tube) are placed. The PEG tube is placed to gravity drainage, and continuous enteral feeding is administered through the J-tube. Ms. Simpson is tolerating tube feeding without difficulty, and mucoid gastric secretions are draining well. On the second day after admission, gastric drainage decreases. Ms. Simpson begins to vomit stomach contents and becomes anxious.

118. To relieve the vomiting, the nurse's **first** step would be to:
    a. irrigate the PEG tube.
    b. turn off the tube feeding.
    c. administer an anxiolytic medication.
    d. increase the rate of intravenous infusion.

119. The progression of Ms. Simpson's tumor has increased her pain. The physician orders oxycodone controlled-release (OxyContin®) for pain management. Ms. Simpson tells the nurse that she is afraid to take the medication because she has heard it is "very addictive." The nurse's best response is:
    a. "Only patients with addictive personalities can become addicted to this medication. Don't worry—it won't happen to you."
    b. "We have physicians trained to handle addictions. Don't worry—if you become addicted, we will help you to recover."
    c. "We will only give you a small dose so that we don't completely relieve your pain, and your chances of addiction are lower. Don't worry—you'll be OK."
    d. "We will carefully monitor the amount you receive and titrate it to control your pain. Don't worry—you'll be safe."

The next three questions pertain to the following scenario.

Arthur Shriver, age 42, is admitted to the medical unit with severe chest pain. A complete cardiac workup is negative, but an esophagogastroduodenoscopy (EGD) confirms gastroesophageal reflux disease (GERD).

120. Mr. Shriver tells the nurse that his chest pain is typically worse after he lies down to sleep at night. The nurse recommends:
    a. eating only a light snack at bedtime.
    b. raising the head of his bed.
    c. using fewer pillows to sleep.
    d. drinking a glass of red wine at bedtime.

121. While teaching Mr. Shriver about his newly prescribed proton pump inhibitor esomeprazole (Nexium®), the nurse instructs him to take the medication:
    a. 1 hour before bedtime.
    b. within 30 minutes of onset of symptoms.
    c. 1 hour before breakfast.
    d. within 30 minutes after eating aggravating foods.

122. Mr. Shriver states, "I can't believe I have GERD. I'll have to avoid all desserts because they will worsen my symptoms." The nurse responds, "Only some desserts aggravate symptoms. You might want to try:
    a. peppermint candies."
    b. apple crumb pie."
    c. chocolate truffles."
    d. citrus fruit cheesecake."

The following are individual questions.

123. A 21-year-old female is diagnosed with Crohn's disease. When teaching her about the disease, the nurse includes the importance of avoiding:
    a. sulfasalazine (Azulfidine®).
    b. vitamin B12.
    c. folic acid.
    d. ibuprofen (Motrin®).

124. In general health screening, the nurse should recognize which patient as at greatest risk for development of gallbladder disease?
    a. 32-year-old man on corticosteroid therapy
    b. 18-year-old woman with anorexia nervosa
    c. 60-year-old woman on estrogen replacement therapy
    d. 40-year-old man with alcoholism

125. Following incisional cholecystectomy, the nurse will monitor the patient's T-tube for:
    a. gastric secretions.
    b. mucoid drainage.
    c. bile drainage.
    d. exocrine secretions.

The next four questions pertain to the following scenario.

Gregory Cavanaugh, age 32, is admitted to the surgical unit following laparoscopic gastroplasty for weight loss. Mr. Cavanaugh weighs 643 pounds.

126. When Mr. Cavanaugh asks about the changes in his stomach, the nurse tells him that his stomach is now the size of:
    a. a football.
    b. an egg.
    c. a softball.
    d. an orange.

127. The nurse knows that leakage at the staple line is a possible complication of Mr. Cavanaugh's surgery. If leakage is suspected, the surgeon is most likely to confirm the integrity of the staple line by ordering a/an:
    a. esophagogastroduodenoscopy (EGD).
    b. abdominal CT scan.
    c. barium swallow study.
    d. gastrograffin study.

128. The nurse recognizes which of the following as a sign of dumping syndrome following gastroplasty?
    a. Constipation
    b. Ileus
    c. Nausea
    d. Bradycardia

129. Because the altered gastrointestinal tract can place Mr. Cavanaugh at risk for malnutrition after discharge, the nurse recommends:
    a. rapid progression to a regular diet.
    b. frequent high-calorie snacks.
    c. daily chewable multivitamins.
    d. broccoli and other nutrient-dense vegetables.

The following are individual questions.

130. The nurse recognizes that the patient experiencing hepatic failure should follow which diet?
    a. Low carbohydrate
    b. No fat
    c. No salt
    d. Low protein

131. The nurse identifies ascites as a complication of cirrhosis that results from:
    a. decreased antidiuretic hormone (ADH).
    b. increased aldosterone secretion.
    c. decreased flow of hepatic lymph.
    d. increased serum oncotic pressure.

132. A 72-year-old male is hospitalized with "coffee ground" emesis of unknown cause. The patient's family is very anxious about the source of bleeding. The nurse informs them that the "gold standard" for diagnosis and treatment of gastrointestinal bleeding is:
    a. angiography.
    b. gastric analysis.
    c. barium contrast studies.
    d. endoscopy.

133. The focus of nursing care for the patient with hepatic encephalopathy is on assisting with measures to reduce the formation of:
    a. urea.
    b. ammonia.
    c. creatinine.
    d. alkaline phosphatase.

134. To evaluate disease progression and reduce the risk of complications from Crohn's disease, the nurse reminds the patient about the importance of regularly scheduled
    a. colonoscopy.
    b. sigmoidoscopy.
    c. defacography.
    d. anorectal manometry.

135. Recognizing that the waist-hip ratio is used to assess body fat distribution, the nurse knows that which of the following measures is associated with increased health risk in women?
    a. 0.2
    b. 0.4
    c. 0.6
    d. 0.8

The following is an individual item.

136. A patient in a women's health clinic has been diagnosed recently with endometriosis. In providing patient education, the nurse should discuss which of the following about this condition?
    a. Endometrial tissue appears outside the lining of the uterine cavity.
    b. Endometriosis is an acute, subacute, or recurrent infection of the oviducts and ovaries, with adjacent tissue involvement.
    c. Endometriosis is caused in part by abnormalities inside or outside the tunica vaginalis that causes excruciating pain.
    d. Biopsy of endometrial tissue reveals a neoplasm in about 20% of women over age 35.

The next three questions pertain to the following scenario.

Charles Manning, age 64, is seen in the clinic with complaint of impotence (also known as erectile dysfunction [ED]). He is open about how his impotence interferes with his self-esteem, relationship with his wife, and overall sense of well-being.

137. What diagnostic tests or procedures can the nurse anticipate to confirm this condition?
    a. Complete blood count and basic metabolic profile
    b. Vascular studies
    c. Digital rectal exam and prostate-specific antigen
    d. Bone density studies

138. In taking the patient's history, the nurse obtains a complete list of medications that Mr. Manning currently takes. Which of the following may cause drug-induced erectile dysfunction?
    a. Lisinopril (Prinivil®) and amitriptyline (Elavil®)
    b. Metformin (Glucophage®) and cephalexin (Keflex®)
    c. Diclofenac (Voltaren®) and esomeprazole (Nexium®)
    d. Dicyclomine (Bentyl®) and pseudoephedrine (Sudafed®)

139. Mr. Manning receives a prescription for sildenafil (Viagra®), an oral medication for treatment of ED. What statement by the patient would indicate he understands the nurse's instructions related to this medication?
    a. "I must take Viagra every morning and can repeat it later in the day if sexual activity is planned."
    b. "I may need to change my eyeglass prescription after 6 months on Viagra."
    c. "I will have to stop taking Viagra if I'm ever prescribed nitroglycerin for angina."
    d. "I may have an erection that lasts longer than 4 hours after I've taken Viagra."

The following are individual items.

140. The nurse identifies which of the following as possible clinical manifestations in a woman who is **perimenopausal?**
    a. Stress incontinence and osteoporosis.
    b. Irregular menses and vasomotor instability.
    c. Vasomotor instability and atrophy of genitourinary tissue with decreased support.
    d. Cessation of menses and osteoporosis.

141. The nurse is caring for a patient admitted with a suspected ectopic pregnancy. The nurse reviews the patient's subjective and objective data. What would suggest that the patient had a ruptured fallopian tube?
    a. Increased hematocrit and bradycardia
    b. Abrupt cessation of pain and vaginal drainage
    c. Cool, clammy skin and decreased blood pressure
    d. Doubling hCG levels and vague abdominal pain

The next two questions pertain to the following scenario.

Ashley Meadows, age 23, is a patient on the medical unit. She offers a new complaint of pain and burning with urination. A urine culture is sent to the laboratory, and she is diagnosed with a urinary tract infection. The physician orders appropriate medications, which are administered to the patient.

142. Ms. Meadows calls from the bathroom 6 hours later. When the nurse enters the room, the patient anxiously reports that her urine is now orange-red in color. The nurse reassures Ms. Cook that the color is a common side effect of which medication?
    a. Oxybutynin (Ditropan®)
    b. Ciprofloxacin (Cipro®)
    c. Trimethoprim/sulfamethoxazole (Bactrim®)
    d. Phenazopyridine (Pyridium®)

143. To help prevent future urinary tract infections, the nurse instructs Ms. Meadows to:
    a. pat dry after urinating to prevent irritation.
    b. wear cotton underwear to prevent moisture.
    c. urinate forcefully to clear bacteria from the tract.
    d. urinate before sexual intercourse to limit transmission.

The next four questions pertain to the following scenario.

Robert Ciccone, age 67, is admitted to the surgical unit after a transurethral resection of the prostate (TURP) for benign prostatic hypertrophy (BPH). His continuous bladder irrigation (CBI) is infusing, and 2,600 cc remain in the bag. The urine bag had been emptied in the postanesthesia care area.

144. Near the end of the shift, the nurse notes that the CBI bag contains 1,200 cc and the urine output bag contains 2,025 cc. The nurse records Mr. Ciccone's true urine output for the shift as:
   a. 1,025 cc.
   b. 825 cc.
   c. 625 cc.
   d. 425 cc.

145. The nurse also notes that Mr. Ciccone's urine output is dark red. Over the next hour, his urine output begins to decrease. Per protocol, the nurse increases the CBI rate; however, output continues to decrease. The nurse notifies the physician and anticipates an order to:
   a. insert a new three-way urinary catheter.
   b. irrigate the urinary catheter with a syringe.
   c. decrease the balloon tension on the urinary catheter.
   d. decrease traction on the urinary catheter.

146. The next day, the nurse enters Mr. Ciccone's room and finds him crying. He tells the nurse that he is upset because he will now be impotent. Which of the following is the nurse's best response?
   a. "Only a percentage of patients experience persistent impotence."
   b. "Impotence is not a potential side effect of this surgery."
   c. "The impotence only lasts a few weeks."
   d. "The impotence is intermittent."

147. Mr. Ciccone prepares for discharge. In the discharge instructions, the nurse teaches the patient the importance of:
   a. bladder isometrics.
   b. opioid analgesic avoidance.
   c. ureteral irrigation.
   d. increased fluid intake.

The next three questions pertain to the following scenario

Jessica Morales, age 34, is admitted with right flank pain due to two large renal calculi. Admission orders include intravenous (IV) fluids at 125 ml/hr and morphine sulfate 2 mg IV every 2 hours as needed for pain. The nurse administers the analgesic in response to Ms. Morales' complaint of pain rated 6 on a 0 to 10 pain intensity scale. Within 30 minutes, the patient rates her pain as 3 and describes it as "tolerable."

148. Two hours later, Ms. Morales calls the nurse with a complaint of recurrent pain, now 8 on a 0 to 10 scale. The nurse administers morphine per order, but the pain remains unchanged, and the patient points to her groin rather than her flank. The nurse calls the physician because of concern about:
   a. analgesic rebound.
   b. hernia reduction.
   c. acute obstruction.
   d. drug-seeking behavior.

149. The following day, one of Ms. Morales' stones is removed through a percutaneous nephroscope. A percutaneous nephrostomy tube is left in place overnight. The nurse assesses the patient for complications and plans to notify the physician immediately for:
   a. flank mass.
   b. hematuria.
   c. flank pain.
   d. nausea.

150. Stone analysis reveals an oxalate stone. To prevent future oxalate stones, the nurse instructs Ms. Morales to avoid:
   a. white bread.
   b. spinach.
   c. liver.
   d. yogurt.

The next three questions pertain to the following scenario.

Claudia Alexander, age 46, is admitted with a complaint of vague abdominal pain and nausea. She has performed peritoneal dialysis at home for 6 months and is now diagnosed with peritonitis. Her chronic renal failure is due to hypertension.

151. During the admission assessment, what is the **most important** question the nurse should ask to confirm the patient's diagnosis of peritonitis?
    a. "How frequently do you void each day?"
    b. "Have you noticed any swelling in your feet today?"
    c. "Have you had any shortness of breath recently?"
    d. "What is the color of your drainage after dialysis?"

152. The nurse would expect the physician to monitor the patient's response to treatment by ordering daily:
    a. blood urea nitrogen (BUN) and creatinine.
    b. effluent cell count and differential.
    c. serum white blood count with differential.
    d. electrolytes.

153. Which of the following interventions is of highest priority in preventing the reoccurrence of peritonitis in Ms. Alexander?
    a. Teach her the manifestations of peritonitis.
    b. Use sterile technique when connecting dialysate bags.
    c. Give antibiotics and heparin as ordered by the physician.
    d. Advise the patient to shower every day.

The next three questions pertain to the following scenario.

Charles Cox, age 38, is scheduled for a left nephrectomy. He was diagnosed with polycystic kidney disease (PKD) 4 years ago, and the disease has been unresponsive to treatment.

154. Which of the following manifestations would confirm that Mr. Cox is exhibiting polycystic kidney disease?
    a. Hypertension, abdominal/flank pain, constipation, hematuria
    b. Hypertension, increased abdominal girth, diarrhea, cloudy urine
    c. Hypotension, abdominal/flank pain, cloudy urine, constipation
    d. Hypotension, increased abdominal girth, diarrhea, hematuria

155. During the first 8 hours after surgery, Mr. Cox develops apparent urinary drainage on his incision dressing. The nurse notes that the surgeon does not have any "call" orders about this occurrence. The nurse should:
    a. call the surgeon immediately because the patient may have an anastomotic leak.
    b. change the dressing to see if the patient has dehisced or eviscerated his incision.
    c. reinforce the dressing because this is an expected finding after this procedure.
    d. monitor the patient's intake and output every 30 minutes until the drainage stops.

156. Mr. Cox tells the nurse that he heard somewhere he could have "passed this problem" to his children. How should the nurse respond?
    a. "Polycystic disease may develop in any of your children."
    b. "Polycystic disease is not a genetic problem."
    c. "Polycystic disease is transmitted from male to male. You said you have all girls."
    d. "Polycystic disease skips a generation, so you don't have to worry about your children."

The next three questions pertain to the following scenario.

Regina Greer, age 57, was diagnosed recently with chronic renal failure due to diabetes. She comes into the outpatient surgery center for placement of an arteriovenous (AV) graft.

157. Ms. Greer asks, "How long will it be before the graft can be used for dialysis?" How should the nurse respond?
    a. "You will be going to the dialysis center from the hospital for your first treatment."
    b. "As soon as you develop a bruit and thrill in your graft, you will start dialysis."
    c. "The graft will only be used if you ever need hemodialysis."
    d. "It takes about 2 to 4 weeks for your graft to be ready for dialysis."

158. Ms. Greer is admitted to the hospital 3 days after placement of the AV graft. Her serum potassium is 6.6 mEq/Liter, and the physician plans to do emergent dialysis. The nurse understands that vascular access will be obtained by:
    a. using the patient's AV graft.
    b. inserting a temporary vascular access device.
    c. inserting a permanent catheter.
    d. initiating peritoneal dialysis.

159. Ms. Greer previously received dietary counseling about avoiding foods that may increase her potassium level. The nurse asks the patient what she had for lunch today. Which of the following would indicate that Ms. Greer needs reinforcement for her diet education?
    a. BLT sandwich with cantaloupe and honeydew for dessert
    b. Turkey and cheese sandwich with grapes
    c. Chicken and noodle soup and a bologna sandwich
    d. Chef salad with garlic toast

The following are individual questions.

160. A patient has a left nephrostomy tube due to renal cancer. The drainage is very thick. The physician orders the tube to be irrigated with 30 cc of sterile water every 8 hours. The nurse decides that this order needs clarification because standards indicate that a nephrostomy tube should be irrigated with:
    a. 5 cc of sterile saline every 8 hours.
    b. 30 cc of sterile saline every 8 hours.
    c. 5 cc of sterile water once a day.
    d. 30 cc of sterile saline once a day.

161. A patient underwent a ureteroenterocutaneous diversion procedure 2 days earlier. When assessing the patient, the nurse would expect to find a:
    a. red, edematous stoma.
    b. pink, flat stoma.
    c. bluish, edematous stoma.
    d. red, flat stoma.

The next two questions pertain to the following scenario.

Rhonda Webster, age 39, is scheduled to undergo laparoscopic tubal sterilization.

162. After the procedure, Ms. Webster reports pain on her left side near her chest and shoulder. The nurse identifies this as **most likely** due to:
    a. myocardial infarction.
    b. musculoskeletal pain from perioperative postioning.
    c. phantom pain.
    d. referred pain from gaseous irritation.

163. The nurse should include which of the following in Ms. Webster's discharge instructions?
    a. "Tub baths are permissible and may improve any postoperative discomfort."
    b. "Limit caffeine for the next 24 to 48 hours."
    c. "Avoid sexual intercourse until after your postoperative appointment with your physician."
    d. "Remain on bed rest for the next 48 to 72 hours."

The next two questions pertain to the following scenario.

Elizabeth Guinyard, age 45, is scheduled for total abdominal hysterectomy. She is accompanied to the hospital by her husband, who is present when the nurse provides preoperative instructions.

164. Mr. Guinyard comments, "Liz is so active. It's going to be hard for her to stay in bed for the next few days." The nurse realizes that further teaching is needed because patients who undergo hysterectomy:
    a. begin ambulation immediately after surgery.
    b. generally go home the day of surgery.
    c. are at increased risk for decubitus ulcers.
    d. are at increased risk for thromboembolism.

165. After her surgery, the nurse finds Ms. Guinyard crying. The nurse knows that body image disturbance is common after hysterectomy and can best support the patient by:
    a. referring her to outpatient counseling.
    b. including her husband in discussions.
    c. allowing the patient privacy.
    d. providing printed material about other women's experiences.

The next two questions pertain to the following scenario.

The nurse has admitted a 32-year-old patient with Guillain Barré Syndrome.

166. The nurse understands that the **primary** concern in the daily management of the patient with Guillain Barré Syndrome involves:
    a. maintaining the airway.
    b. maintaining adequate blood pressure.
    c. preventing pressure ulcers.
    d. preventing injuries from seizures.

167. When discussing Guillain Barré Syndrome with the patient, the nurse explains that:
    a. weakness usually plateaus and begins improving after 4 weeks.
    b. sensory functions return before muscle strength in 90% of patients.
    c. residual weakness and absent reflexes usually persist in the ankles and feet for 6 months.
    d. respiratory therapy is usually required for 6 months from onset of symptoms.

The next three questions pertain to the following scenario.

John Bouknight, age 62, has a 5-year history of Parkinson's disease (PD).

168. As Mr. Bouknight ambulates with a walker, he stops and tells the nurse his legs "feel as if they are glued to the floor." The nurse recognizes this as the "freezing of gait," a common development in PD that requires the nurse to:
    a. report the finding to the physical therapist.
    b. initiate fall risk procedures for the patient.
    c. call the physician to discuss medication side effects.
    d. initiate relaxation training to assist the patient with ambulation.

169. The nurse observes Mr. Bouknight become agitated and non-directable, picking at things in the air. The nurse identifies this as:
    a. a usual symptom in PD and secludes the patient in a quiet area.
    b. most likely due to overdosing of levodopa (Sinemet®) and calls the physician.
    c. indicative of a seizure and lowers the patient slowly to the floor.
    d. suggestive of dehydration and provides additional oral fluids.

170. In talking with a nursing orientee about Mr. Bouknight's diagnosis, the nurse identifies which of the following as the **most frequent** cause of death in patients with PD?
    a. Pneumonia
    b. Injuries from falls
    c. Injuries other than falls
    d. Venous thromboemolism

The following are individual questions.

171. A patient experiences acute alterations in mental status. Based on laboratory results, the nurse suspects the change is due to which electrolyte disturbance?
    a. Hyperkalemia
    b. Hypokalemia
    c. Hyponatremia
    d. Hypernatremia

172. A patient has orders for medications in all the following classes. Which class is **most likely** to be associated with altered mental status?
    a. Calcium channel blocker
    b. Beta blocker
    c. Diuretic
    d. Antiarrhythmic

173. A 72-year-old woman experiences her first generalized (tonic-clonic) seizure and is hospitalized. Her family asks the nurse why the patient would have a seizure. The nurse's response is based on the understanding that the most common co-morbid diagnosis associated with onset of seizures in older adults is:
    a. Alzheimer's disease.
    b. Pick's disease.
    c. acute stroke.
    d. acute infection.

The next two questions pertain to the following scenario.

Maria Steria, age 30, is admitted to the medical unit with complaints of intermittent weakness, loss of sensation in her lower extremities, and vision changes. Her provisional diagnosis is multiple sclerosis (MS).

174. Ms. Steria tells the nurse that she has become more depressed due to her frequent urinary incontinence. She describes an inability to hold any urine and states, "It just seems to come out without warning." Based upon knowledge of the most common cause of urinary incontinence in patients with MS, the nurse suggests the patient eliminate which of the following from her diet?
    a. Milk
    b. Orange juice
    c. Coffee
    d. Red wine

175. The nurse recognizes that different types of incontinence may occur with MS. To differentiate incontinence due to flaccid or spastic bladder, the nurse will:
    a. request a physician order for oxybutynin (Ditropan® XL).
    b. perform a bladder scan after each patient void.
    c. have the patient increase her intake of water.
    d. collect the patient's urine via straight catheterization for a urinalysis.

The following are individual questions.

176. A malnourished patient is admitted to the medical unit with acute alcohol withdrawal syndrome. The patient's confusion and lack of muscle coordination are consistent with Wernicke's encephalopathy. The nurse knows that the nerve damage associated with this complication is caused by lack of:
    a. niacin.
    b. thiamine.
    c. riboflavin.
    d. pyridoxine.

177. A patient with osteoporosis is taking teriparatide (Forteo®) and asks the nurse how the medication works. The nurse's response is based on understanding that teriparatide:
    a. slows the activity of osteoclasts.
    b. stimulates the activity of osteoblasts.
    c. stimulates the activity of osteocytes.
    d. slows the activity of osteophytes.

178. Following application of a long-leg cast, the nurse will assess sensation and motion in the patient's digits. Numbness and tingling at the tip of the great toe may indicate compromise of which nerve?
    a. Peroneal
    b. Sural
    c. Sapphenous
    d. Median

179. A patient arrives on the surgical unit following kyphoplasty of thoracic vertebrae 11 and 12 (T11 and T12). The nurse will institute spine precautions that require:
    a. forward bending exercises to strengthen the spine.
    b. logrolling for bed mobility.
    c. sitting for frequent periods in a recliner.
    d. rotational exercises to increase spine flexibility.

The next three questions pertain to the following scenario.

Alfred Cowan, age 62, is hit by a car when crossing the street. After he is transported to the Emergency Department, X-ray confirms a comminuted fracture of the midshaft of the right femur. There is also evidence of a healed fracture of the right tibia. Mr. Cowan undergoes open reduction and internal fixation of the right femur, and is transferred to the surgical unit. His postoperative orders include morphine sulfate by patient-controlled analgesia (PCA) pump.

180. Compared to analgesia administered by intramuscular injection, the nurse knows that PCA has the advantage of:
    a. allowing for individual titration of analgesia.
    b. decreasing the amount of analgesia that can be administered.
    c. reducing the need for nursing assessment of the patient's pain.
    d. permitting family members to administer analgesia.

181. The nurse recognizes Mr. Cowan is at increased risk for fat embolism due to:
    a. his age.
    b. the fracture site.
    c. previous fracture of the same extremity.
    d. the use of internal fixation.

182. The nurse will monitor Mr. Cowan for early signs and symptoms of fat embolism syndrome (FES), which include:
    a. hypothermia.
    b. anuria.
    c. restlessness.
    d. bradycardia.

The next seven questions pertain to the following scenario.

Margaritte Chiu, age 64, has osteoarthritis and is scheduled for right total hip arthroplasty. Ms. Chiu comes to the ambulatory care area of the hospital for her preoperative visit 2 days before the surgery.

183. Ms. Chiu makes all of the following statements to the nurse. Which one definitely indicates the need for further investigation?
    a. "I'm getting so stiff that I can barely move around."
    b. "Every night I have a little glass of wine before bedtime."
    c. "The arthritis in my shoulder has been bothering me this week."
    d. "I had a nasty tooth pulled yesterday."

184. Ms. Chiu has given two units of blood for her own use after surgery. What is one advantage of preoperative autologous blood donation?
    a. Shortened transfusion time
    b. Less risk of postoperative infection
    c. Decreased likelihood of transfusion reaction
    d. Need for a lower dose of anticoagulant

Ms. Chiu undergoes right total hip arthroplasty with a posterolateral approach. After recovery in the postanesthesia care area, she is transferred to the surgical unit. Orders include morphine sulfate by patient-controlled analgesia (PCA) pump.

185. Which of these observations made by the nurse would indicate that Ms. Chiu's right lower extremity was correctly positioned after surgery?
    a. Leg is in neutral position.
    b. Leg is in adducted position.
    c. Hip is flexed 90 degrees.
    d. Hip is internally rotated.

186. The nursing assistant reports Ms. Chiu's complaint of pain to the nurse. The nurse takes all of the following actions. Which action should the nurse take **first**?
    a. Administer the dosage prescribed for "breakthrough" pain.
    b. Determine if the PCA pump is working properly.
    c. Examine Ms. Chiu's operative site.
    d. Assess the site and intensity of Ms. Chiu's pain.

187. Ms. Chiu would have a positive Homan's sign if she described calf pain when her:
    a. knee is pressed against the bed and her leg is extended.
    b. foot is dorsiflexed and her leg is extended.
    c. foot is laterally rotated and her knee is flexed.
    d. knee is flexed and her foot is internally rotated.

188. As Ms. Chiu becomes more independent in her mobility, the nurse coaches her on continued attention to hip precautions. Which of the following activities might cause dislocation of the patient's hip prosthesis?
    a. Standing with right toes pointed outward
    b. Sitting on a 21-inch toilet seat
    c. Picking up a book that has fallen from the nightstand
    d. Pulling up the bed sheets with a long-handled reacher

189. Ms. Chiu has been receiving enoxaparin (Lovenox®) to decrease her risk of blood clots. What will the nurse instruct Ms. Chiu about correct use of enoxaparin after discharge?
    a. Heparin can be substituted for enoxaparin if cost is an issue.
    b. Inject the medication in the anterolateral abdomen.
    c. Purge air from the syringe before administration.
    d. Gently rub the injection site to disperse the medication.

The next four questions pertain to the following scenario.

Sandra Miller, age 74, is admitted to the medical unit with a recent history of right-sided facial droop, limited movement of the right extremities, and slurred speech. The physician diagnoses a cerebrovascular accident (CVA).

190. The nurse recognizes Ms. Miller's symptoms as **most indicative** of damage to the:
    a. temporal lobe.
    b. left side of the brain.
    c. right side of the brain.
    d. occipital lobe.

191. Ms. Miller's daughter tells the nurse that her mother frequently cries during their visits. The nurse's best explanation would be:
    a. "Your mother is in an unfamiliar place and really misses you."
    b. "Your mother needs to re-learn appropriate social behavior."
    c. "The patient becomes extremely self-absorbed after a stroke."
    d. "Emotional responses may be unpredictable after a stroke."

192. Ms. Miller is allowed nothing by mouth until evaluation by the speech therapist. The nurse realizes this is due to Ms. Miller's increased risk for:
    a. bronchitis.
    b. pleural effusion.
    c. aspiration.
    d. pulmonary contusion.

193. Ms. Miller's physician prescribes clopidogrel (Plavix®) 75 mg by mouth daily. During use of this medication, the nurse will monitor Ms. Miller for which side effect?
    a. Atrial fibrillation
    b. Prolonged bleeding
    c. Blurred vision
    d. Anorexia

The following are individual items.

194. A patient with a hip fracture is placed in 5 pounds of Buck's traction, and surgery is scheduled for the next morning. The nurse knows the Buck's traction is used to:
    a. minimize muscle spasm.
    b. increase blood flow to fracture fragments.
    c. decrease the risk of thrombosis.
    d. maximize the patient's bed mobility.

195. A patient is placed in a continuous passive motion (CPM) machine following total knee arthroplasty. To ensure effective use of the machine, the nurse will instruct the nursing assistant to:
    a. place the patient in the machine only after visitors have left for the day.
    b. elevate the foot of the patient's bed at least 30 degrees.
    c. raise the head of the patient's bed no more than 15 degrees.
    d. keep the patient in the machine during meals to maximize use.

Hematologic, Immunologic, and Integumentary   **Questions 196-213**

The following are individual items.

196. The nurse provides self-care instructions related to thrombocytopenia for a patient with leukemia. What response from the patient would indicate the nurse needed to reinforce instructions?
    a. "I need to shave with an electric razor only."
    b. "I should not blow my nose forcefully."
    c. "I can take aspirin if I have pain or a headache."
    d. "I need to get help when getting out of bed if I feel weak."

197. A 56-year-old female recently received chemotherapy for breast cancer and now has an absolute neutrophil count of 1450 cells/mm3. The nurse recognizes that the patient now:
    a. is predisposed to infection.
    b. has the potential to bleed easily.
    c. will be fatigued and short of breath.
    d. may have cardiac rhythm changes.

198. A patient with a stage IV pressure ulcer on the sacrum has been receiving treatment with moist dressing changes three times daily. On initial assessment, the nurse observes full-thickness tissue loss surrounded by pink healing tissue with no bone, tendon, or muscle exposed. How will the nurse identify this wound?
    a. Reversed stage IV pressure ulcer, now stage III
    b. Granulating stage IV pressure ulcer
    c. Healing stage II pressure ulcer
    d. Unstageable pressure ulcer

199. A patient's wound is being managed with vacuum assisted closure (VAC®). During the night, the machine malfunctions and must be stopped, and a replacement is unavailable until morning. When deciding how to proceed, the nurse must understand that the current occlusive wound VAC dressing should be:
    a. left in place as it is keeping the wound covered.
    b. replaced with a moist dressing.
    c. replaced with a dry sterile dressing.
    d. removed and replaced with a new wound VAC dressing.

The next three questions pertain to the following scenario.

Ruth Zaiger, age 28, is admitted to the medical unit after an exacerbation of systemic lupus erythematosus (SLE). She was diagnosed with SLE 10 years ago.

200. Ms. Zaiger is scheduled to undergo plasmapheresis for the first time and asks the nurse why this procedure is used for individuals with SLE. The nurse explains that plasmapheresis is used to:
    a. remove blood components that have been damaged by autoantibodies.
    b. replace damaged autoantibodies with whole blood.
    c. exchange the patient's plasma with antinuclear antibodies for a substitute fluid.
    d. replace the patient's T lymphocytes with antinuclear antibodies.

201. Ms. Zaiger is receiving intravenous methylprednisolone (Solumedrol®). During **short-term** treatment with methylprednisolone, the nurse will most appropriately monitor the patient's:
    a. weight.
    b. liver function tests.
    c. serum glucose.
    d. respirations.

202. Which statement by Ms. Zaiger would indicate her understanding of effects of the disease?
   a. "Lying in the summer sun helps to dry the rash on my face."
   b. "My husband and I plan to have a child when the lupus is controlled."
   c. "I know I just have to work through the joint pain."
   d. "I can't get the pneumonia vaccine because of the lupus."

The next three questions pertain to the following scenario.

Marcia Chapel, age 32, is admitted to the medical unit with pneumonia. Ms. Chapel was diagnosed with acquired immunodeficiency syndrome (AIDS) last year. She had a positive HIV-antibody test 6 years ago but refused to begin antiretroviral therapy because of medication side effects.

203. The nurse knows that a diagnosis of AIDS is made when an HIV-infected patient has:
   a. vaginal candidiasis.
   b. a CD4:CD8 ratio of less than 2:1.
   c. Hodgkin's lymphoma.
   d. a CD4+ T cell count below 200/microliter.

204. Ms. Chapel agrees to start antiretroviral therapy. The nurse correctly explains the goal of therapy as:
   a. decreasing the patient's risk for opportunistic infection.
   b. increasing the patient's immunosuppressant ability.
   c. decreasing the patient's viral load.
   d. increasing the patient's tolerance.

205. What is the most appropriate action for the nurse to take to help Ms. Chapel follow her antiretroviral treatment regimen after discharge?
   a. Assess the patient's lifestyle for adherence cues.
   b. Volunteer to create a drug pillbox for the first week.
   c. Give the patient a videotape and brochure about treatment.
   d. Tell the patient that the side effects will go away within weeks.

The following are individual items.

206. Assessment leads the nurse to believe that a newly admitted patient may be severely anemic. Findings that suggest anemia include:
   a. bradycardia.
   b. increased appetite.
   c. decreased pulse pressure.
   d. jaundice.

207. A patient admitted for sickle cell crisis suddenly develops fever, chest pain, cough, and dyspnea. The nurse recognizes this complication as:
   a. acute chest syndrome.
   b. autosplenectomy.
   c. hemochromatosis.
   d. pulmonary hypertension.

208. In differentiating Hodgkin's disease and non-Hodgkin's lymphoma, the nurse knows that:
   a. non-Hodgkin's lymphoma requires a staging laparotomy.
   b. Hodgkin's disease only affects young adults.
   c. non-Hodgkin's lymphoma is treated solely with radiation therapy.
   d. Hodgkin's disease is considered potentially curable.

209. A patient with paraplegia and multiple pressure ulcers is being discharged home to the care of family members. In teaching the family about care of pressure ulcers, the nurse will instruct them to:
   a. reposition the chair-bound patient every hour.
   b. use a doughnut cushion for pressure relief in the wheelchair.
   c. limit the patient's fluids to avoid urinary incontinence.
   d. institute a low-calorie diet for the patient's weight control.

210. A patient is diaphoretic and frequently incontinent of urine. The nurse recognizes the patient is at risk for which skin disorder?
   a. Tinea pedis
   b. Candidiasis
   c. Verruca vulgaris
   d. Impetigo

211. In managing pain for a burn patient, the nurse knows that treatment will be most effective when:
   a. painful dressing changes are delayed until pain is completely relieved.
   b. the nurse provides opioid analgesics on a set schedule.
   c. visualization and relaxation are the first-line interventions for pain management.
   d. the patient has as much control as possible over pain management strategies.

212. The patient has a skin tear on the right forearm. For this dry, noninfected wound, the nurse's best choice will be which of the following dressings?
   a. Alginate dressing such as Sorbsan®
   b. Hydrocolloid dressing such as Tegasorb™
   c. Antimicrobial dressing such as Acticoat™
   d. Polyurethane dressing such as OpSite®

213. A patient is having an acute rejection of a transplanted organ. The nurse will expect to administer which of the following drugs?
    a. Tacrolimus (Prograf®)
    b. Muromonab-CD3 (Orthoclone OKT® 3)
    c. Cyclosporine (Sandimmune®)
    d. Mycophenolate mofetil (CellCept®)

The following are individual questions.

214. A patient with acromegaly asks the nurse about the cause of this disorder. The nurse's response is based on knowledge that acromegaly develops due to pathology of the:
    a. pituitary gland.
    b. adrenal gland.
    c. thyroid gland.
    d. pineal gland.

215. In a patient diagnosed with syndrome of inappropriate anti-diuretic hormone (SIADH), the nurse would expect laboratory findings to include which of the following?
    a. Hypocalcemia
    b. K+ 4.8 mEq/L
    c. Na+ 110 mEq/L
    d. Hypermagnesemia

216. The nurse recognizes that electrolyte abnormalities in the patient with SIADH may present as:
    a. double vision.
    b. abdominal cramps.
    c. tachycardia.
    d. tachypnea.

217. A 30-year-old female has been diagnosed with Cushing's syndrome. The nurse knows that she is **most likely** to exhibit which triad of symptoms?
    a. Hypertension, hirsutism, polyuria
    b. Hypotension, anemia, polyuria
    c. Menstrual irregularities, hypoglycemia, obesity
    d. Hyperkalemia, menstrual irregularities, obesity

218. The nurse knows that which urine test would be used for diagnosis of pheochromocytoma?
    a. pH
    b. Osmolality
    c. Metanephrines
    d. Culture and sensitivity

219. A nursing plan of care for the patient with hypoparathyroidism would include teaching the patient about which of the following?
    a. Physical restrictions
    b. Limited dietary potassium
    c. Phosphorus supplements
    d. Rebreathing techniques

220. A 74-year-old male is admitted to the surgical unit following a total thyroidectomy. What additional equipment should the nurse include in the patient's room set up?
    a. Chest tube insertion tray
    b. Central line insertion tray
    c. Tracheostomy tray
    d. Thoracotomy tray

221. A 62-year-old female is admitted to the medical unit. When considered with other physical findings, the nurse suspects the patient has Grave's disease because of the presence of:
    a. dry eyes.
    b. exophthalmos.
    c. pigeon chest.
    d. hirsutism.

The next two questions pertain to the following scenario.

222. Bernard Webb, age 44, is transferred to the surgical unit following total thyroidectomy. The nurse's postoperative monitoring is based on recognition of which of the following as the **most critical** potential complication?
    a. Seizures
    b. Neck stiffness
    c. Bleeding
    d. Pain

223. Two days after surgery, Mr. Webb complains of muscle cramps and tingling in his lips. The nurse will call the physician to share these findings, which are **most likely** the result of:
   a. damage to the parathyroid glands during surgery.
   b. residual effects of general anesthesia.
   c. decreasing serum magnesium following surgery.
   d. cervical spine compromise.

The following are individual questions.

224. The nurse is teaching a patient with a new diagnosis of diabetes mellitus about disease management. Among the "survival skills" that the nurse should identify is:
   a. weight loss.
   b. eliminating sugar from the diet.
   c. self-monitoring of blood glucose.
   d. limited physical activity.

225. A patient diagnosed with diabetes insipidus asks the nurse about the cause of other increased urinary output. The nurse's response is based on understanding that the polyuria is due to:
   a. decreased adrenocorticoid secretion.
   b. decreased antidiuretic hormone secretion.
   c. increased adrenocorticoid secretion.
   d. increased antidurietic hormone secretion.

226. The nurse knows that the older adult who experiences thyroid problems requires additional monitoring because the:
   a. size of the thyroid gland increases with advancing age.
   b. amount of thyroid secretions increase with advancing age.
   c. basal ganglion response decreases with advancing age.
   d. basal metabolic rate decreases with advancing age.

227. The nurse knows that the risk of diabetic foot ulcers is greatly increased in the patient with:
   a. neuromegaly.
   b. neuropathy.
   c. neurogenesis.
   d. neuroblastosis.

228. The patient with type 2 diabetes mellitus tells the nurse he also takes several herbal supplements. The nurse identifies which of the following supplements as **decreasing** the antidiabetic effects of the patient's oral agent?
   a. St. John's wort
   b. Ginseng
   c. Bee pollen
   d. Garlic

The next three questions pertain to the following scenario.

229. Douglas Maddox, age 20, presents with a blood glucose of 816 mg/dl. The nurse suspects diabetic ketoacidosis (DKA) rather than hyperosmolar hyperglycemic nonketotic syndrome (HHNS) because of the assessment finding of:
   a. peripheral edema.
   b. polyuria.
   c. rapid, deep respirations.
   d. petechiae.

230. The physician starts Mr. Maddox on rapid-acting insulin. When monitoring the patient, the nurse knows that the onset of rapid-acting insulin is:
   a. 15 minutes.
   b. 30 minutes.
   c. 45 minutes.
   d. 60 minutes.

231. Orders for Mr. Maddox also included the oral antidiabetic glyburide (Micronase®). The nurse's discussion of the new medication with the patient is based on knowledge that it acts by:
   a. slowing absorption of carbohydrates.
   b. increasing absorption of carbohydrates.
   c. stimulating insulin secretion.
   d. limiting insulin secretion.

The following are individual questions.

232. When asked about the action of glargine insulin (Lantus®), the nurse informs the patient that it:
   a. peaks 4 hours after administration.
   b. peaks 6 hours after administration.
   c. peaks 8 hours after administration.
   d. has no peak action.

233. Which of the following statements should the nurse include in teaching a patient to self-administer glargine insulin?
   a. Do not mix glargine insulin with any other insulin.
   b. Discard unused glargine insulin 14 days after opening the vial.
   c. Glargine insulin is cloudy in appearance.
   d. Use the same syringe with other insulin to save supplies.

234. The nurse recognizes the potential for secondary diabetes in a patient with a diagnosis of:
   a. Hashimoto's thyroiditis.
   b. hypopituitarism.
   c. hyperthyroidism.
   d. Addison's disease.

235. The nurse understands that symptoms of hyperosmolar hyperglycemic nonketotic syndrome (HHNS) may include:
    a. somnolence.
    b. anuria.
    c. arterial pH <7.2.
    d. bradycardia.

236. In caring for a culturally diverse patient population, the nurse knows that the highest incidence of diabetes occurs in which of the following groups?
    a. Native Americans.
    b. African Americans.
    c. Hispanics.
    d. Asians.

237. A patient is diagnosed with insulin resistance syndrome. The nurse recognizes that this patient is also at **greatest** risk for:
    a. renal insufficiency.
    b. cardiovascular disease.
    c. liver failure.
    d. pancreatic cancer.

238. The nurse knows that the timing of insulin administration in relation to meals is important. The nurse will administer a **rapid-acting** insulin:
    a. 45 minutes before the meal.
    b. with the meal.
    c. 15 minutes after the meal.
    d. 1 hour after the meal.

239. The patient who is most ikely to develop hyperosmolar hyperglycemic nonketotic syndrome (HHNS) is the one who is taking long-term:
    a. vitamin K.
    b. corticosteroids.
    c. antihypertensive medication.
    d. warfarin (Coumadin®).

240. A patient with type 2 diabetes mellitus is being treated with insulin and a sulfonylurea. The nurse knows the patient is at increased risk for:
    a. hypoglycemia.
    b. HHNS.
    c. DKA.
    d. insulin resistance.

241. To decrease the risk for development of diabetic neuropathy, the nurse will encourage the patient to:
    a. drink 8 to 10 glasses of water daily.
    b. eliminate alcohol.
    c. decrease consumption of red meat.
    d. stop smoking.

242. A patient is taking acarbose (Precose®), an oral agent for diabetes mellitus management. The nurse will monitor the long-term effectiveness of acarbose by checking the patient's:
    a. fasting blood glucose.
    b. 2-hour postprandial blood glucose.
    c. hemoglobin A1C.
    d. Somogyi effect.

243. A nurse discusses the use of an insulin pump with a patient with type 1 diabetes mellitus. The nurse knows that the pump will deliver:
    a. intermittent doses of insulin in response to the patient's blood glucose.
    b. intermittent doses of insulin when the patient presses a trigger.
    c. continuous doses of insulin during the patient's waking hours.
    d. continuous doses of insulin around-the-clock as a basal rate.

At the conclusion of each answer below will be a cross-referenced code identifying the item's content based on the medical-surgical nursing certification examination blueprint: physiological system and domain of nursing practice. The physiological system will be identified first, the domain second. For example, questions about the gastrointestinal system in the helping domain will be noted as "GH." A detailed description of the domains is included on pages 4-5.

Phys Domain	GI	Pulm	Cardio	Diab/Endo	GU/Ren/ Repro	MS/Neur	Hem/Im/ Integ
Help	GH	PH	CH	DH	GUH	MH	HH
Teach	GT	PT	CT	DT	GUT	MT	HT
Diag	GD	PD	CD	DD	GUD	MD	HD
Admin	GA	PA	CA	DA	GUA	MA	HA
Change	GC	PC	CC	DC	GUC	MC	HC
Monitor	GM	PM	CM	DM	GUM	MM	HM
Org	GO	PO	CO	DO	GUO	MO	HO

1. Correct answer – C. Hypercarbic respiratory failure occurs when conditions cause a reduction in minute volume or an increase in physiologic dead space (for example, COPD [including bronchitis], asthma, exacerbation of underlying neuromuscular disease). Hypoxic respiratory failure results from an insult to the pulmonary tissues (such as pneumonia, ARDS, pulmonary contusion). (PD)

2. Correct answer – B. Cardiotoxicity can develop from a cumulative drug effect. Altering the dose scheduling of doxorubicin to include frequent lower doses has resulted in reduction of cardiotoxity without compromise of antitumor effects. (PD)

3. Correct answer – A. Pulmonary function tests are used to identify and quantify abnormalities in respiratory function, including three general patterns of abnormality: obstructive, restrictive, and mixed. (PM)

4. Correct answer – C. The skin test should be read 48 to 72 hours after it has been administered. (PM)

5. Correct answer – B. Assess pH; less than 7.35 = acidosis. Assess pCO_2; greater than 45 = respiratory acidosis. (PD)

6. Correct answer – C. Common acute risks of tracheostomy include bleeding, airway loss, damage to adjacent structures, and failure of the chosen technique to achieve successful airway placement. (PM)

7. Correct answer – B. O_2 therapy should be started immediately, with administration monitored by pulse oximetry to keep SpO_2 greater than 90%. Aerosolized medications will be given by neublizer or metered-dose inhaler every 20 minutes for 1 hour. Systemic conticosteroids will be indicated if the initial response to the bronchodilator is insufficient. (PC)

8. Correct answer – D. Because people with CF can have malabsorption resulting in low bone mineral content, they are at risk for osteopenia. (PT)

9. Correct answer – B. Hypotension can occur when giving etoposide. The patient should be instructed to call the nurse immediately if he or she feels dizzy or faint during administration of the drug. (PT)

10. Correct answer – A. Oral care for the patient with mucositis should be performed at least before and after each meal and at bedtime. A saline solution of 1 tsp. of salt in 1 liter of water is an effective cleansing agent; 1 tsp. of sodium bicarbonate may be added to the oral care solution to decrease odor, alleviate pain, and dissolve mucin. (PT)

11. Correct answer – B. Walking programs are a way of keeping the patient active. Walking programs have been found to lessen anxiety and fatigue. (PH)

12. Correct answer – B. Risk factors for community-acquired pneumonia include diabetes, cardiovascular disorders, alcohol abuse, and immunosuppression. Other factors do not significantly affect pneumonia risk. (PD)

13. Correct answer – C. The patient's complaint of chest tightness may suggest a pneumothorax. Other answers are normal for a patient with pneumonia. (PC)

14. Correct answer – B. Manufacturer's guidelines call for intramuscular injection of the pneumococcal vaccine, preferably into the mid-lateral thigh or deltoid. (PA)

15. Correct answer – C. Tuberculosis is caused by *Mycobacterium tuberculosis*, an acid-fast organism. (PA)

16. Correct answer – A. Ibuprofen is a nonsteroidal anti-inflammatory drug that may increase bleeding risk for an invasive procedure, such as bronchoscopy. Other routine medications that do not increase risk for bleeding can be taken with a sip of water on the morning of the procedure. (PA)

17. Correct answer – C. Tuberculosis is spread when organisms remain suspended in air currents in the room after being dispersed via a cough, laugh, or sneeze from the infected person. Airborne precautions, including the use of a microparticulate mask, are necessary for health care providers. (PA)

18. Correct answer – D. Factors, agents, or situations that may affect readings, limit precision, or limit the performance or application of a pulse oximeter include skin pigmentation, motion artifact, abnormal hemoglobins (primarily carboxyhemoglobin [COHb] and methemoglobin [metHb]), intravascular dyes, exposure of measuring probe to ambient light during measurement, low perfusion states, and nail polish or nail coverings with finger probe. (PD)

19. Correct answer – B. The Heimlich valve is a one-way valve used instead of water-seal drainage for treatment of an uncomplicated pneumothorax or hemothorax. (PA)

20. Correct answer – A. Following a bronchoscopy, the patient is kept NPO until return of the gag reflex. (PD)

21. Correct answer – B. Isoniazid is the drug of choice for treating latent tuberculosis. (PA)

22. Correct answer – D. Pressure changes in the pleural space cause fluctuations in the water level in the water seal chamber of a chest tube. (PA)

23. Correct answer – D. *Haemophilus influenzae* is a common cause of community-acquired pneumonia in the elderly. (PD)

24. Correct answer – C. Leukotriene modifiers prevent bronchoconstriction and have an anti-inflammatory effect. (PA)

25. Correct answer – B. The patient should be reminded to rinse his or her mouth after inhalation to reduce the risk of yeast infection. The drug is not used to treat asthma attacks. The inhaler should be used for no more than 1 month after opening; the patient should keep track of doses and discard the inhaler after 120 doses, even if medicine still appears to be in the device. Special tests may be needed to determine if the patient with diabetes can safely use the inhaler. (PT)

26. Correct answer – D. When fever occurs in a neutropenic patient, it is generally assumed to be caused by infection and requires immediate attention because the immunocompromised patient lacks normal protective mechanisms. (PD)

27. Correct answer – A. Peak expiratory flow rate (PEFR) is normally 600 L/minute, but with an asthma exacerbation, it may be as low as 100 to 150 L/minute. A SaO_2 of 88% and FEV1 of 80% of predicted **[Dottie – predicted what?]** can be seen in mild-to-moderate asthma. Interstitial infiltrates may be an indicator of infection. (PD)

28. Correct answer – D. Pulse oximetry is inaccurate if the probe is loose, or in the presence of poor circulation, nail polish, or dark skin pigmentation. (PM)

29. Correct answer – D. Cromolyn is particularly effective in preventing exercise-induced asthma when taken 10 to 20 minutes before exercise. (PT)

30. Correct answer – B. Chronic bronchitis is diagnosed after a chronic productive cough is present for 3 months in 2 successive years. (PD)

31. Correct answer – A. Alpha-antitrypsin deficiency is a known genetic abnormality that leads to COPD/emphysema. (PD)

32. Correct answer – C. The major purpose of PEEP is to improve oxygenation while decreasing the risk of oxygen toxicity. (PA)

33. Correct answer – D. A correctly positioned ET tube is associated with symmetrical chest movement. (PM)

34. Correct answer – A. Drop precautions are indicated for the patient with meningococcal pneumonia. The patient with varicella is placed on airborn isolation. The immunocompromised adult with RSV would be placed on contact precautions. The patient with pneumococcal pneumonia only requires use of standard precautions. (PA)

35. Correct answer – C. A V/Q scan is primarily used to diagnose a pulmonary embolus. (PD)

36. Correct answer – A. Respiratory acidosis with hypercapnia and hypoxemia are characteristic of late-stage COPD. (PD)

37. Correct answer – C. Pursed-lip breathing prolongs exhalation and prevents bronchiolar collapse and air trapping. Diaphragmatic breathing emphasizes the use of the diaphragm to maximize inhalation and slow respirations. Inhaling or exhaling quickly has no value. (PT)

38. Correct answer – D. A non-rebreather mask delivers a FiO_2 of 100%. (PA)

39. Correct answer – B. Diminished/absent breath sounds indicate a decrease in air movement as the result of fatigue and the inability to generate enough muscle force to ventilate. This is an ominous sign. (PD)

40. Correct answer – A. A pulmonary angiogram involves the injection of an iodine-based radiopaque dye into the pulmonary artery; therefore, iodine and shellfish allergies should be assessed before injection. There is no need for the patient to be NPO or to withhold medication except for metformin (Glucophage®) or other medication as determined by the physician. (PA)

41. Correct answer – C. To promote self-efficacy, it is important to understand and teach according to the patient's needs. (PT)

42. Correct answer – B. Apnea during the sleep cycle causes hypoxemia and hypercapnia, stimulating ventilation and awakening the patient. This frequent awakening can result in morning headaches, insomnia, and excessive daytime sleepiness. The degree of mattress firmness and a history of asthma or cough are not relevant factors. (PD)

43. Correct answer – C. Increased respiratory rate and hyperventilation create a respiratory alkalosis with increased pH and decreased $PaCO_2$, followed by hypoxemia. (PD)

44. Correct answer – A. A yellow zone reading indicates that the patient is getting worse; quick-relief medications should be used. Peak flow meter readings are done optimally when the patient gets up and before he or she goes to sleep, so the bulky meter does not need to be carried at all times. The peak flow meter measures the ability to empty the lungs of air, not the amount of air inhaled. (PT)

45. Correct answer – D. The patient experiencing an acute asthma exacerbation will be fearful and anxious. It is important for the nurse to stay with the patient for ongoing assessment and to provide a calm environment. Helping the patient breathe with pursed lips will facilitate the expiration of trapped air and help the patient regain control of his or her breathing. (PC)

46. Correct answer – D. According to the Centers for Disease Control and Prevention, a person who developed Guillain-Barré syndrome within 6 weeks of previous influenza vaccination should not receive additional vaccine. Severe allergy to chicken eggs is also a potential contraindication. Reaction to pneumococcal vaccine and contact with a 50-year-old are not considerations. (PT)

47. Correct answer – D. Although other methods may work, the most successful programs for smoking cessation combine behavioral approaches with pharmacological interventions. (PH)

48. Correct answer – D. Eating is an effort for the patient with COPD. The patient frequently does not eat due to fatigue, dyspnea, and difficulty holding the breath to swallow. Foods that require excessive chewing can cause exhaustion. A low-carbohydrate diet is recommended if the patient is hypercapnic because carbohydrates are metabolized into carbon dioxide. Cold foods give less of a feeling of fullness than hot foods. (PA)

49. Correct answer – A. The destruction of alveolar walls and the loss of lung elasticity lead to air trapping in the alveoli of the patient with emphysema. (PT)

50. Correct answer – D. Pleuritic (knife-like) chest pain is a typical symptom of pulmonary embolus. Additional symptoms include shortness of breath or coughing up blood. Knife-like chest pain is not associated with the other conditions. (PD)

51. Correct answer – D. Because beta-blockers dilate the peripheral arterial system, sudden changes in position can cause dizziness, lightheadedness, or syncope. These responses are most prominent when beginning the drug. To promote safety, especially for older persons, nurses should teach those taking beta-blockers to change positions very slowly. The drug should be taken with food to increase absorption; there is no need to increase fluid intake, which could worsen the hypertension; vision is not affected by this drug. (CT)

52. Correct answer – D. Fast food is usually high in sodium, which contributes to hypertension. Daily walking is a positive activity and should be encouraged. One glass of wine or beer daily is considered moderate intake and is not contraindicated with hypertension. Body mass index of 18 to 25 is normal and would not contribute to hypertension. (CD)

53. Correct answer – A. A disturbing potential side effect of beta-blockers is impotence. This response by the nurse depersonalizes the sexual problem and allows the patient a comfortable opening to discuss his concerns. Answer B makes the assumption that fatigue is the problem without further questioning. Answer C sounds probing, and answer D has a lecturing tone without acknowledging the patient's concerns. (CA)

54. Correct answer – B. Unstable angina is characterized by unpredictable intensity, frequency, or duration of chest pain. It often occurs with minimal activity or at rest. Unstable angina does not alter ventricular contractility, nor does it produce Q-waves on an ECG, as does MI. (CM)

55. Correct answer – C. Rapid ventricular heart rates result in shortened filling time for the ventricles. Less filling time causes a reduction in ventricular preload (filling pressure/volume) and a decrease in cardiac output. This is more likely to occur in older patients who have decreased ventricular compliance. Rapid heart rate does not cause narrowing of coronary arteries and does not cause pulmonary emboli. Shortness of breath can occur, but this would be secondary to the altered cardiac output. (CC)

56. Correct answer – A. The patient should understand that pain unrelieved by 3 sublingual nitroglycerin tablets taken 5 minutes apart is likely due to an acute coronary syndrome (ACS) and that she should seek help immediately. Nitroglycerine will not prevent an MI. The other choices are facts that the patient should know but are not the most important. (CT)

57. Correct answer – C. Morphine relieves chest pain, which in turn decreases cardiac contractility and oxygen consumption by the myocardium. These actions improve cardiac output. None of the other drugs listed improve both anxiety and cardiac output. (CA)

58. Correct answer – B. Dysrhythmias are the most common complication of acute MI. Cardiogenic shock, cardiac tamponade, and valvular rupture are possible complications of MI but are not common. (CM)

59. Correct answer – C. Mild temperature elevation with MI is due to a systemic inflammatory response associated with myocardial injury and resolves within a few days. It does not indicate infection, dehydration, or pericarditis. (CD)

60. Correct answer – B. Immediately following an MI, activity is usually limited to self-care activities and bathroom privileges. Limiting activity during the first 1 to 2 days decreases cardiac workload and oxygen consumption when the myocardium is most vulnerable to complications. (CM)

61. Correct answer – D. A cardiac catheterization can be used to measure intracardiac pressures and oxygen levels in various parts of the heart, as well as cardiac output. With injection of dye and X-ray visualization, the chambers of the heart can be outlined and heart motion observed. In addition, the coronary arteries can be visualized, and any obstruction to the blood flow can be seen. (CT)

62. Correct answer – C. Patients who are sensitive to iodine or shellfish often have an allergic reaction to the dye used in cardiac catheterization. (CM)

63. Correct answer – D. Smoking causes vasoconstriction that further impedes blood flow. The patient should be instructed to avoid smoking and be counseled to begin a smoking cessation program. (CT)

64. Correct answer – A. The patient should be advised that pain not relieved by three sublingual tablets over a 15-minute period may indicate an acute MI or severe coronary insufficiency. It is important to advise the patient to contact a physician immediately or have someone take the patient directly to the emergency room. (CT)

65. Correct answer – B. An anterior infarction primarily damages the left ventricle. The symptoms of heart failure are related to the left side of the heart. Shortness of breath, palpitation, and weakness are symptoms that the patient should report immediately. (CT)

66. Correct answer – A. In heart failure, the compensatory mechanisms cause the retention of fluid and sodium. Intake and output have to be monitored closely, along with daily weight. The nurse should limit family visits only if the patient's condition worsens in response to the increased activity. (CA)

67. Correct answer – B. Anorexia is the most common early indicator of toxicity. (CC)

68. Correct answer – D. Amiodarone, cyclosporine, diltiazem, and erythromycin are drugs that may increase serum digitalis concentration. Rifampicin, neomycin, cholestyramine, colestipol, sulfasalazine, and metoclopramide are drugs that decrease the digitalis concentration. (CA)

69. Correct answer – C. A cornerstone of treatment for CHF is frequent weights, preferably daily. Every patient should have a calculated target weight. Weight gain of 3-5 pounds per week may signal the need for a change in therapy and should prompt a call to the physician. (CH)

70. Correct answer – B. A compensatory mechanism in heart failure is the retention of sodium and water, along with the inability of the kidneys to excrete sodium. Sodium intake should be restricted to 2 to 3 grams/day. (CA)

71. Correct answer – C. Right-sided heart failure can result from primary pulmonary hypertension. Symptoms include distended neck veins, dependent edema, and hepatic engorgement. Conversely, symptoms of left-sided heart failure include dyspnea, crackles, cool extremities, and weak peripheral pulses. (CD)

72. Correct answer – C. Troponin levels provide the important diagnostic criteria for myocardial infarction. Typically, troponin is done 2 or 3 times during a 12 to 16-hour period. (CD)

73. Correct answer – D. Treating pain with opioid analgesics is a priority of care for the patient with chest pain. (CA)

74. Correct answer – A. MIDCABG surgery is limited to those patients with single vessel left ascending artery disease. (CD)

75. Correct answer – A. Heart sounds in severe forms of congestive heart failure are manifested by crackles in the lungs. The pulmonic component of the second heart sound tends to be summated, and an S3 gallop is commonly present. In left-sided heart failure, the low blood pressure results from low cardiac output; thus heart rate increases as a compensatory response. Ascites is a clinical finding of right-sided heart failure. Fever is not associated with heart failure. (CD)

76. Correct answer – B. Patients with permanent pacemakers and their families should be taught how to take the pulse. (CT)

77. Correct answer – C. One of the complications of severe hypertension is hypertensive heart disease, which includes coronary artery disease that can manifest itself as angina and be a precursor for myocardial infarction. Other cardiac complications of severe hypertension include left ventricular hypertrophy and heart failure. (CD)

78. Correct answer – B. Patients should be told not to discontinue antihypertensive drugs abruptly because withdrawal may cause a severe hypertensive reaction. (CT)

79. Correct answer – B. Telmisartan contains the diuretic hydrochlorothiazide, so the patient should ensure the doctor is aware of any other diuretic he is currently taking. Lithium should not be taken with telmisartan. No interaction has been demonstrated with acetaminophen. The drug is taken once daily. (CT)

80. Correct answer – C. Telmisartan is an angiotensin II receptor blocker (ARB). (CA)

81. Correct answer – D. Digitalis is given to treat atrial fibrillation, diuretics to decrease preload, and angiotensin-converting enzyme (ACE) inhibitors to decrease afterload for the patient with cardiomyopathy. (CA)

82. Correct answer – C. ACE inhibitors such as enalapril are used in dilated cardiomyopathy to decrease peripheral blood pressure (afterload). (CA)

83. Correct answer – C. Defibrillation is the most effective treatment for ventricular fibrillation. (CA)

84. Correct answer – D. Following AMI, the patient without contraindications will be placed on a beta-adrenergic blocker. Carvedilol is the only listed medication from this class. (CH)

85. Correct answer – B. Valvular disease increases the risk of developing infective endocarditis, with organism entry occurring through dental work, surgical procedures, or other breaks in skin integrity. (CD)

86. Correct answer – C. Maintaining circulation by increasing fluid volume and keeping the patient NPO to decrease the production of pancreatic enzymes is the appropriate action. Though pain management is a vital intervention for patients with pancreatitis, increased pancreatic secretions would not be a goal of care. Serum calcium levels may already be decreased in pancreatitis so the nurse would not manage fluid hydration in order to decrease these levels. Patients with pancreatitis often have glucosuria and hyperglycemia; steroids will increase the likelihood that these conditions will develop and are not recommended in the treatment of acute pancreatitis. (GM)

87. Correct answer – B. Laboratory tests may demonstrate a marked elevation in the white blood cell count with a left shift to immature forms. Serum creatinine is likely to be increased and albumin decreased in this disorder. Platelets are not affected. (GD)

88. Correct answer – B. MAP = [(2 x diastolic)+systolic] / 3 MAP is a combined measure for organ perfusion. Usual range is 70 to 110. A MAP of 60 is needed to perfuse coronary arteries, brain, and kidneys. Many patients will develop multi-organ failure with a MAP less than 60. (GC)

89. Correct answer – C. HBV is spread by having sex with an infected person, as well as through blood transfusions or needle sharing by IV drug users. Hepatitis A is contracted through fecal contamination and eating raw shellfish. (GD)

90. Correct answer – A. Ascites and GI bleeding (such as tarry stools) are symptoms of portal hypertension. Other symptoms include decreased platelets and decreased white blood cell count. (GC)

91. Correct answer – B. Symptoms are those of decreased brain function, especially reduced alertness and confusion. In the earliest stages, subtle changes appear in logical thinking, personality, and behavior. The person's mood may change, and judgment may be impaired. Normal sleep patterns may be disturbed. At any stage of encephalopathy, the person's breath may have a musty sweet odor. As the disorder progresses, the hands cannot be held steady when the person stretches out the arms, resulting in a crude flapping motion of the hands (asterixis). Also, the person

usually becomes drowsy and confused, and movements and speech become sluggish. Disorientation is common. Uncommonly, a person with encephalopathy becomes agitated and excited. Seizures are also uncommon. (GD)

92. Correct answer – C. Only increased fluids and a laxative promote/aid in the expelling of the barium. (GA)

93. Correct answer – D. Substernal pain that worsens with positioning is typical of gastroesophageal reflux disease (GERD). Peptic ulcer disease is generally accompanied more by abdominal complaints. Gastric cancer is generally painless unless widespread. Duodenal ulcer pain is usually not positional. (GD)

94. Correct answer – A. Peppermint and caraway oil are the most widely used herbal products for relieving symptoms of dyspepsia. Saw palmetto is used by patients with benign prostatic hyperplasia. Black cohosh is believed to relieve perimenopausal symptoms, such as hot flashes. (GT)

95. Correct answer – B. Caffeine-containing beverages (coffee, tea, and cola drinks) and decaffeinated coffee cause increased gastric acid production but may be taken in moderation at or near mealtime, if tolerated. Eat three small meals and three snacks evenly spaced throughout the day to avoid periods of hunger or overeating. Eat slowly and chew foods well. Avoid eating within 3 hours before bedtime. Bedtime snacks can cause gastric acid secretion during the night. (GT)

96. Correct answer – D. In acute GI bleeding, vasomotor stability is the most sensitive indicator. Changes in heart rate and blood pressure of 20 beats or 20 mm Hg systolic blood pressure indicate a loss of 15% to 20% of the total volume. Hemoglobin and hematocrit values do not change for 8 to 20 hours after the bleeding begins. Oxygen saturation gives information about the percentage of hemoglobin that is saturated with oxygen and is not an indicator of blood loss. Patients losing gastric contents along with blood will develop metabolic alkalosis. (GM)

97. Correct answer – C. The nurse should not irrigate or move the nasogastric tube to avoid disrupting the internal suture line of the stomach. All other choices are generally expected postoperative care measures. (GA)

98. Correct answer – B. Appropriate site selection should include the shape and condition of the skin in order to avoid stoma complications. (GM)

99. Correct answer – A. The nurse can provide answers to the patient's questions without referring him to the surgeon. Male impotence is not a common occurrence after ostomy. (GT)

100. Correct answer – C. Skin exposure to stool can be a major problem for the patient with an ostomy. (GT)

101. Correct answer – B. The ileostomy patient can easily become dehydrated and must be carefully monitored. (GA)

102. Correct answer – D. Medications in tablet form may not be readily absorbed by the patient with an ileostomy. Chewable or liquid forms are more immediately available for absorption in the shortened gastrointestinal tract. (GA)

103. Correct answer – C. Because most water is reabsorbed from the colon, the patient who has an ileostomy will have somewhat liquid stools. (GT)

104. Correct answer – A. General guidelines for nutrition after ileostomy include eating slowly and chewing food thoroughly to facilitate digestion. (GT)

105. Correct answer – D. By changing the pouch before meals or when the ostomy is inactive, the patient has less chance of experiencing elimination from the stoma during the change. (GT)

106. Correct answer – A. Colonoscopy is not routinely included in IBD work-up because of the need for vigorous bowel prep and sedation. (GD)

107. Correct answer – C. Crohn's disease, not ulcerative colitis, carries the greater risk for stricture due to intestinal wall thickening and formation of scar tissue. Diet is not linked to disease development. The pain of Crohn's disease is most often in the right lower quadrant, mimicking appendicitis, because that is the location of the terminal ileus. Sulfasalazine rather than methotrexate commonly is prescribed for inflammation; other drugs include those from the 5-ASA drug group, such as mesalamine (Asacol®, Pentasa®). (GT)

108. Correct answer – B. Bowel rest and elemental diet are ordered because they place no demands on the large bowel. (GD)

109. Correct answer – B. Most bleeding ulcers are related to the presence of *Helicobacter pylori* or drug use, especially aspirin and aspirin-containing products (salicylates). Severe retching and vomiting are associated with esophageal bleeding. Spicy foods do not cause ulcers. (GT)

110. Correct answer – A. Some patients experience less pain by assuming positions that flex the trunk and draw the knees up to the abdomen. (GH)

111. Correct answer – B. Nasogastric tube insertion has been associated with increased incidence of sinus infection due to the tube pathway. The tube creates an abnormal pathway for bacteria between the GI tract and the sinus. (GA)

112. Correct answer – D. Gastric secretions are rich in postassium. Both emesis and nasogastric output contribute to the loss of potassium. (GA)

113. Correct answer – C. Low residue diets contain soluble fiber, which moves easily through the GI tract and does not become lodged in narrow areas. (GT)

114. Correct answer – A. A nasogastric tube is never repositioned by the registered nurse in the gastric resection patient. Flushing with saline is the standard of care. Dextrose is unnecessary and may cause dumping syndrome. (GA)

115. Correct answer – D. The nurse should allow the patient to share her concerns and express her feelings in a nonjudgmental environment. (GH)

116. Correct answer – B. Third spacing is a common postoperative complication. Tachycardia, hypotension, and low urine output are key symptoms. (GD)

117. Correct answer – C. Small frequent meals prevent overfilling the stomach, and thus, prevent rapid emptying. Fluids should not be taken with meals, and high carbohydrate diets should be avoided; both contribute to dumping. (GT)

118. Correct answer – A. The mucoid content of the gastric secretions contributes to tube clogging. Irrigating the tube will minimize clogging and promote good flow. (GA)

119. Correct answer – D. Pain management is an essential element of patient care. The nurse should allay patient fears, anxieties, and misconceptions while appropriately treating the patient's pain. (GH)

120. Correct answer – B. The head of the bed should be elevated to permit gravity to assist with the appropriate flow of gastric secretions and to minimize regurgitation into the esophagus. (GM)

121. Correct answer – C. Esomeprazole works best on an empty stomach and should be taken an hour before meals. (GT)

122. Correct answer – B. Spicy foods, cocoa, mints, and fatty foods typically increase symptoms of GERD. Apple crumb pie is the least offensive. (GT)

123. Correct answer – D. Ibuprofen may cause bleeding of the Crohn's ulcers. The other medications may be required for treatment. (GT)

124. Correct answer – C. Incidence of cholelithiasis is higher in women, multiparous women, and persons over 40 years of age. Postmenopausal women on estrogen replacement therapy are at greater risk of having gallbladder disease than are women who are taking birth control pills. Other factors that seem to increase the occurrence of the disease are a sedentary lifestyle, a familial tendency, and obesity. (GD)

125. Correct answer – C. Following incisional cholecystectomy, the patient may have a T tube to allow bile drainage. (GA)

126. Correct answer – B. Following gastroplasty, the patient's stomach is approximately the size of an egg. (GT)

127. Correct answer – D. To verify that no leakage occurs into the abdominal cavity from the staple line, the surgeon will order a gastrograffin study. (GD)

128. Correct answer – C. Nausea and vomiting, abdominal bloating, diarrhea, and vasomotor symptoms (flushing, increased heart rate, sweating, lightheadedness) can be indicative of dumping syndrome. (GA)

129. Correct answer – C. A daily multivitamin in chewable or liquid form is recommended. The patient will remain on a pureed diet for approximately 6 weeks. The patient should avoid high-calorie snacks and hard vegetables, such as broccoli and cauliflower. (GT)

130. Correct answer – D. The patient experiencing hepatic failure should follow a low-protein diet (limited to 20 grams/day at onset of severe hepatic failure). Protein is broken down to ammonia, which cannot be cleared by the failing liver. (GA)

131. Correct answer – B. Ascites is linked to increased aldosterone secretion, which stimulates decreased renal blood flow; metabolism of aldosterone also is impaired in liver disease. Serum oncotic pressure is decreased because of loss of albumin into the peritoneal cavity, and excessive serum levels of ADH result in impaired water excretion. Flow of hepatic lymph is increased from the cirrhotic liver. (GD)

132. Correct answer – D. Endoscopy is the best method for identifying the source of an upper GI bleed and also for many treatment modalities. Examples of treatment using endoscopy are cautery of the bleeding vessels, constriction of the vessels by rubber banding, and embolization of the bleeding vessels with an autologous clot or a clotting substance, such as Gelfoam®. (GT)

133. Correct answer – B. Elevated ammonia is an indicator of advanced liver disease and will affect mental status. (GD)

134. Correct answer – A. Crohn's disease increases the risk of colon cancer. Screening colonoscopy is required to examine the entire colon and rule out cancerous changes. (GT)

135. Correct answer – D. A waist-hip ratio of 0.8 or greater is associated with increased health risk in women. (GD)

136. Correct answer – A. Ectopic endometrial tissue responds to estrogen and progesterone with proliferation and secretion. During menstruation, ectopic tissue bleeds and causes inflammation of the surrounding tissues. Answer B describes pelvic inflammatory disease. Answer C describes testicular torsion, a male reproductive disorder. Answer D applies to uterine leiomyomas, also known as myomas, fibromyomas, and fibroids. (GUD)

137. Correct answer – B. Vascular studies, including penile arteriography, penile blood flow study, and duplex Doppler ultrasound studies, are used to assess penile blood circulation. These studies help assess vascular problems interfering with erection. Blood work that the doctor might order include serum glucose, lipid profile, testosterone, prolactin, and thyroid hormone levels. DRE and PSA tests assess prostate problems. Bone density plays no role in erectile dysfunction. (GUD)

138. Correct answer – A. Risk factors for drug-induced ED include but are not limited to use of alcohol, antihypertensives, caffeine, diuretics, opioids, and tricyclic antidepressants. (GUM)

139. Correct answer – C. Viagra may potentiate the hypotensive effect of nitrates, so the drug is contraindicated for individuals taking nitroglycerin. Viagra should be taken orally about 1 hour before sexual activity but not more than once a day. Vision changes are not expected; blindness is a rare side effect. Priapism (persistent penile erection) is considered a medical emergency. (GUT)

140. Correct answer – B. Hallmarks of the perimenopausal period include vasomotor instability (hot flashes) and irregular menses. Answers A, C, and D are incorrect because they each contain some aspect of menopause. Manifestations of menopause include cessation of menses, occasional vasomotor symptoms, atrophy of genitourinary tissue with decreased support, and osteoporosis. (GUD)

141. Correct answer – C. Vital signs should be monitored closely, along with signs and symptoms of shock. The patient will have increased pain and vaginal bleeding. If tubal rupture occurs, the pain is intense and may be referred to the shoulder as a result of irritation of the diaphragm by blood released into the abdominal cavity. Suspected rupture is treated as an emergency. If the patient is hemorrhaging, her hematocrit would decrease and her heart rate would increase. The pain usually increases, as does the vaginal bleeding. B-hCG levels double in a normal pregnancy, not in an ectopic pregnancy. (GUC)

142. Correct answer – D. Phenazopyridine alters the color of urine. The other medications do not change urine color. (GUT)

143. Correct answer – B. Bacteria thrive in a dark, moist environment. Cotton absorbs moisture and pulls it away from the skin. (GUT)

144. Correct answer – C. 2,600 cc – 1,200 cc = 1,400 cc irrigant used during shift; 2,025 cc in urine bag – 1,400 cc irrigant used = 625 cc true urine output during shift. (GUA)

145. Correct answer – B. Irrigation clears thick blood clots, which may block the drainage tube and lead to low urine output. The nurse would never change the urinary catheter or alter traction on a urinary catheter placed following TURP. (GUD)

146. Correct answer – A. The nurse should clarify misconceptions and provide accurate patient education. (GUH)

147. Correct answer – D. Increasing fluid levels will help keep urine free of blood clots and promote good urinary outflow. (GUT)

148. Correct answer – C. Renal calculi are mobile. Complications of obstruction are noted by a change in a pain location and increased pain that is unresponsive to analgesia. (GUD)

149. Correct answer – A. Flank mass is a sign of hematoma, a serious complication requiring immediate physician notification. (GUC)

150. Correct answer – B. Spinach is high in oxalate. (GUT)

151. Correct answer – D. The primary clinical manifestation of peritonitis is a cloudy peritoneal effluent with white blood cell count over 100 cells/microliter. (GUD)

152. Correct answer – B. See rationale for 151. (GUD)

153. Correct answer – B. The most common cause of peritonitis is connection site contamination. To prevent peritonitis, use meticulous sterile technique when caring for the peritoneal dialysis catheter and connecting or disconnecting the bags. (GUA)

154. Correct answer – A. Key features of PKD are abdominal/flank pain, hypertension, nocturia, increased abdominal girth, constipation, bloody or cloudy urine, and kidney stones. (GUD)

155. Correct answer – C. It is also important to assess for urine drainage on the dressing and estimate the amount. (GUM)

156. Correct answer – A. The patient who has adult polycystic disease often has children by the time the disease is diagnosed. Each child of a parent with polycystic kidney disease has a 50% chance of having the disease. (GUT)

157. Correct answer – D. It takes 2 to 4 weeks for a graft to heal. During this time, the endothelial cells are deposited on the inside of the graft, and these cells help seal the needle puncture site after the dialysis catheter is removed. (GUT)

158. Correct answer – B. In some cases, when temporary vascular access is required quickly, percutaneous cannulation of the subclavian, internal jugular, or femoral vein is performed. (GUA)

159. Correct answer – A. Cantaloupe and honeydew melons are very high in potassium. (GUT)

160. Correct answer – A. No more than 5 cc of sterile saline solution is gently instilled at one time to prevent over-distention of the renal pelvis and renal damage. (GUM)

161. Correct answer – A. A healthy stoma is beefy red and swollen in the immediate postoperative period. (GUD)

162. Correct answer – D. The peritoneal cavity is filled with 3 to 4 liters of carbon dioxide to separate the abdominal wall from the viscera and increase visualization. At the end of the procedure, the carbon dioxide is removed, but referred pain to the shoulder may occur from gaseous irritation of the diaphragm and phrenic nerve. (GUD)

163. Correct answer – C. Discharge instructions include rest for 24 to 48 hours and regular diet with plenty of fluids. Tub baths are discouraged. Sexual activity should not be resumed until after the first postoperative appointment with the surgeon. (GUT)

164. Correct answer – D. Venous pooling and pelvic congestion are concerns after hysterectomy because of the inflammatory response to the trauma of surgery. The risk of thromboembolism is significant. (GUT)

165. Correct answer – B. The nurse should provide opportunities for the patient to express feelings and concerns about the loss of her uterus, and should assess the significant other's concerns and perceptions. The nurse can help the patient and significant other express doubts and resolve concerns. (GUH)

166. Correct answer – A. Respiratory distress, respiratory failure, increased secretions in the airway, and inability to clear secretions are all primary concerns with GBS. The other choices are not primary concerns but could be secondary issues associated with GBS. (MM)

167. Correct answer – C. Weakness plateaus and begins improving after 4 weeks in 90% of patients with GBS. The majority of patients recover to their pre-illness strength and level of activity within months of the illness. Respiratory therapy is only needed during acute hospitalization, before weakness plateaus. The pattern of sensory and motor recovery will vary significantly between patients. (MT)

168. Correct answer – B. Falling and associated fall-risk factors have received little attention in PD research. Approximately 70% of PD patients fall, 13% weekly. Falls result in hip fractures, injuries, hospitalizations, and disability. Longer duration of disease, dyskinesias, freezing of gait, postural instability, increased disability, depression, and weaker proximal lower extremity strength have been identified as fall-risk factors for patients with PD. (MM)

169. Correct answer – B. Psychosis in patients with Parkinson's disease is often drug-induced. It can be managed by decreasing doses of anticholinergics or dopamine agonists and by using the lowest possible dose of levodopa. (MD)

170. Correct answer – A. Due to immobility, pneumonia is the most frequent cause of death. (MT)

171. Correct answer – C. Hyponatremia classically presents with altered mental status as its primary symptom, especially in elders. It is the most frequent electrolyte disturbance seen in U.S. hospitals. (MM)

172. Correct answer – C. Diuretic use (especially furosemide [Lasix®]) can be associated with hyponatremia from loss of electrolytes. (MM)

173. Correct answer – C. Studies of new onset seizures in patients over age 60 have consistently found stroke as the most common co-morbid diagnosis. (MT)

174. Correct answer – C. Detrusor hypercontractility and failure to store syndromes are the most common type of bladder dysfunction in MS. Treatment includes use of behavioral techniques and anticholinergics, and avoiding stimulants, such as coffee and tea. (MT)

175. Correct answer – B. In order to determine whether the incontinence is due to flaccid or spastic bladder, a bladder scan is indicated after each void. This will help the physician determine appropriate medication for the patient. (MD)

176. Correct answer – B. Wernicke's encephalopathy involves damage to multiple nerves in both the central nervous system (brain and spinal cord) and the peripheral nervous system (the rest of the body). It may also include symptoms caused by alcohol withdrawal. The cause is generally attributed to malnutrition, especially lack of vitamin B1 (thiamine), which is common in those with alcoholism. Heavy alcohol use interferes with the break down of thiamine in the body, so even if someone with alcoholism follows a well-balanced diet, most of the thiamine is not absorbed. (MD)

177. Correct answer – B. Teriparatide, unlike bisphosphonates, does not kill the cells that destroy bone (osteoclasts). Instead, it stimulates the bone-builders, known as osteoblasts. (MT)

178. Correct answer – A. The great toe is innervated by the deep peroneal nerve. (MM)

179. Correct answer – B. Twisting and bending should be avoided after spine surgery. Logrolling is used for bed mobility to ensure the patient's torso is moved as a single unit. (MA)

180. Correct answer – A. PCA offers the patient some control over analgesia administration. The pump can be programmed per physician order to administer an individually determined dosage. The nurse still needs to assess the patient's pain on a regular basis. Family members should be discouraged from pushing the button on the PCA pump. (MA)

181. Correct answer – B. Fracture of the pelvis or long bones, such as the femur, greatly increases the patient's risk for fat embolism. (MD)

182. Correct answer – C. Primary symptoms of FES include changes in mental status, increasing respiratory distress, and petecchiae of the skin and mucosa. Initial changes in mental status may be restlessness, somnolence, or confusion, which can then progress to complete loss of consciousness. (MD)

183. Correct answer – D. Dental work releases bacteria into the blood stream that may seed a surgical site and increase the risk of infection. (MD)

184. Correct answer – C. The patient is less likely to react to her own blood than to banked blood received from volunteer donors. (MA)

185. Correct answer – A. The operative leg must be kept in a neutral position, usually with a pillow or wedge in place to maintain it in abduction to decrease the risk of hip dislocation. Flexion of 90 degrees or more and internal rotation also increase the risk of dislocation. (MA)

186. Correct answer – D. The nurse must completely assess the patient's pain first, especially noting if it is increased or in a different location since the first assessment. Results of the assessment will determine the nurse's subsequent actions. (MD)

187. Correct answer – B. Pain on passive stretch of the calf muscles is a positive Homan's sign. This is elicited by having the patient dorsiflex her foot while her leg is fully extended. (MD)

188. Correct answer – C. Bending past 90 degrees at the waist can increase the risk of hip dislocation. The patient should use assistive devices, such as a long-handled reacher, to pick up any items on the floor. All other activities are appropriate. (MA)

189. Correct answer – B. Enoxaparin should be administered between the anterolateral and posterolateral abdomen. The air bubble should not be expelled before medication administration, and the site should not be rubbed (to avoid bruising). Enoxaparin is not interchangeable with unfractionated heparin or other low-molecular weight heparin. (MT)

190. Correct answer – B. Right-sided symptoms typically indicate left-brain damage following CVA. (MD)

191. Correct answer – D. Patients who have had a CVA may have difficulty controlling their emotions, which may be exaggerated or unpredictable and unrelated to surrounding events. (MH)

192. Correct answer – C. Following a CVA, the patient may have swallowing difficulties due to partial paralysis of muscles in the jaw and throat. Aspiration precautions should be implemented until evaluation determines that the patient is able to take food or fluid. (MD)

193. Correct answer – B. Clopidrogel is an anti-platelet drug that decreases the risk of clot formation. The patient who takes it is at increased risk for bleeding episodes and should be carefully monitored. (MA)

194. Correct answer – A. Disabling muscle spasm can occur after hip fracture. Use of Buck's traction provides some immobilization of fracture fragments, thus decreasing the likelihood of spasm in the surrounding muscles. (MA)

195. Correct answer – C. The patient should be in the CPM machine at least 8 hours daily to maximize effects on joint range of motion. The foot of the bed should be locked in extended or flat position. The head of the bed should be no higher than 15 degrees during machine use to avoid placing additional torque on the knee. Because of that, the patient should be out of the machine and upright during meals. The patient can remain in the machine while visitors are present. (MM)

196. Correct answer – C. A patient who has thrombocytopenia needs to avoid any OTC medicines that can prolong clotting, such as aspirin or NSAIDS. All other answers are proper self-care practices for a thrombocytopenic patient. (HT)

197. Correct answer – A. A neutropenic patient is at risk for infections with non-pathogenic organisms that constitute normal body flora, as well as opportunistic pathogens. Answer B describes a patient experiencing thrombocytopenia. Answers C and D describe symptoms for a patient experiencing anemia. (HM)

198. Correct answer – B. Avoid reverse staging a stage III or stage IV pressure ulcer unless required by regulations governing the care setting. Reverse staging implies that the wound has replaced lost muscle and subcutaneous tissue. For example, documenting that a stage IV pressure ulcer is now stage III indicates that the wound bed is now filled with healthy subcutaneous tissue when, in fact, a stage IV pressure ulcer heals by granulation tissue formation, not regeneration of muscle, fat, and dermis. Healing is more appropriately reflected by changes in wound dimension and by notation that the wound is a granulating stage IV pressure ulcer. (HD)

199. Correct answer – B. The wound VAC provides negative pressure, which aids in healing as well as prevents tissue desiccation. If another machine is not available, the most appropriate action is to place a moist dressing over the wound. (HM)

200. Correct answer – C. Plasmapheresis involves the removal of plasma containing components causing or thought to cause disease. The plasma is replaced with a substitute fluid, such as saline or albumin. (HT)

201. Correct answer – C. Corticosteroids tend to affect blood glucose and cholesterol levels, as well as blood pressure. Other side effects, such as weight gain, fluid retention, and infection, are usually seen with **long-term** use of corticosteroids. (HA)

202. Correct answer – B. For the best outcome, pregnancy should be planned when disease activity is minimal. Sun exposure should be limited and sunscreens should be used. The patient should pace and prioritize activities during episodes of joint pain or fatigue. Because the patient is at increased risk for infection, particularly respiratory infection, she should receive a pneumonia vaccination;

however, she should avoid live-virus vaccines when being treated with corticosteroids or cytotoxic agents. (HT)

203. Correct answer – D. According to the Centers for Disease Control and Prevention (CDC), AIDS is diagnosed when an individual develops at least one of these conditions: CD4+ count bellow 200 cells/microliter; development of an opportunistic infection (including candidiasis of the bronchi, trachea, lungs, or esophagus), development of an opportunistic cancer, wasting syndrome, dementia. (HD)

204. Correct answer – C. The goal of antiretroviral therapy is to decrease the patient's viral load, the amount of virus in the blood. (HT)

205. Correct answer – A. Although strategies, such as the pillbox or videotape, may be helpful, the nurse can best offer assistance by learning about the patient's lifestyle and offering tips within the confines of that routine. (HH)

206. Correct answer – D. Severe anemia is diagnosed when hemoglobin is less than 6 grams/dL. Symptoms include tachycardia, anorexia, increased pulse pressure, and jaundice (related to hemolysis). (HD)

207. Correct answer – A. Acute chest syndrome is characterized by fever, chest pain, cough, pulmonary infiltrates, and dyspnea. (HC)

208. Correct answer – D. Radiation therapy can cure 95% of patients with stage I or stage II Hodgkin's disease; treatment advances now enable some stage IIIB and stage IV diseases to be cured with high-dose chemotherapy and bone marrow or peripheral stem cell transplantation. Staging of both Hodgkin's disease and non-Hodgkin's lymphoma is accomplished through peripheral blood analysis, lymph node biopsy, bone marrow examination, and radiologic evaluation. Non-Hodgkin's lymphoma is treated with both chemotherapy and radiation. (HD)

209. Correct answer – A. The chairbound patient should be repositioned every hour; the bed-bound patient at least every 2 hours. Doughnut cushions can create an area of ischemia

and should not be used. The patient should consume 2,000 to 3,000 calories and 2,000 ml of fluid per day to provide calories, protein, and fluids necessary for tissue repair. (HT)

210. Correct answer – B. Candidiasis (yeast infection) frequently develops in warm, moist areas, such as the groin and submammary folds. Tinea pedis is commonly known as athlete's foot. Verruca vulgaris is caused by human papillomavirus. The lesions of impetigo develop as a result of bacterial infection. (HD)

211. Correct answer – D. The most important point to remember about pain management is that the more control the patient has, the more successful the chosen strategies will be. Nonpharmacologic strategies, such as visualization and relaxation, are used as adjuncts to traditional pharmacological treatments. (HH)

212. Correct answer – D. A transparent polyurethane dressing is the most appropriate choice for a dry, noninfected wound. The other listed dressings are used for draining or infected wounds. (HA)

213. Correct answer – B. Muromonab-CD3 is a monoclonal antibody used for the prevention and treatment of acute rejection episodes. The other drugs are immunosuppressant drugs used to prevent a cell-mediated attack against a transplanted organ. (HA)

214. Correct answer – A. The pituitary gland is responsible for growth hormone; any excess due to tumor can cause acromegaly in adults and gigantism in children. (DT)

215. Correct answer – C. A defining characteristic of SIADH is hyponatremia due to sustained released of ADH. Normal serum sodium is approximately 135 to 145 mEq/L. (DM)

216. Correct answer – B. Signs and symptoms of hyponatremia include abdominal cramps. The remaining options are not signs and symptoms of hyponatremia. (DM)

217. Correct answer – A. Hypertension may result from fluid retention due to mineralocorticoid excess. Additionally, the female patient with Cushing's syn-

drome may exhibit truncal or generalized obesity and "moon facies," hirsutism, menstrual disorders, hypertension, and hypokalemia. (DD)

218. Correct answer – C. The level of metanephrines is elevated due to results of metabolic products of epinephrine and norepinephrine. (DD)

219. Correct answer – D. Rebreathing may partially alleviate acute neuromuscular symptoms related to hypocalcemia (such as generalized muscle cramps, mild tetany). The patient who is able to cooperate should be instructed to breathe in and out of a paper bag or breathing mask. This reduces CO_2 excretion from the lungs, increases serum carbonic acid, and lowers pH. (DT)

220. Correct answer – C. A tracheostomy tray should be available because of the patient's risk of respiratory distress related to swelling of the operative site. An emergency tracheostomy would be indicated. (DA)

221. Correct answer – B. Classic symptoms of Grave's disease include an enlarged thyroid gland (goiter), nervousness, heat intolerance, weight loss, sweating, diarrhea, tremors, palpitations, and exophthalmos (swelling of the tissue behind the eyeballs causing protrusion of the eyeball). The patient may have increased tearing and hair loss as well. (DD)

222. Correct answer – C. Postoperative bleeding can be a devastating complication of thyroid surgery. An unrecognized or rapidly expanding hematoma can cause airway compromise and asphyxiation. Pain would be present, but bleeding is more crucial. (DM)

223. Correct answer – A. Damage to the parathyroid glands is a complication during thyroidectomy due to their proximity to the thyroid gland. Tingling and muscle cramps are manifestations due to the loss of parathyroid hormone that controls calcium. (DC)

224. Correct answer – C. Self-monitoring of blood glucose is the foundation of successful disease management for the patient with diabetes mellitus. (DT)

225. Correct answer – B. Decrease in ADH secretion would prompt polyuria, with output of 3 liters/day or more. (DT)

226. Correct answer – D. Decreased peripheral metabolism is one age-related change that occurs in the endocrine system. The older adult also experiences decreased secretion of antidiuretic hormone (ADH), decreased gonad function, and decreased glucose tolerance. (DM)

227. Correct answer – B. Diabetic neuropathy is nerve damage that occurs because of metabolic derangements associated with diabetes mellitus. The most common type is sensory neuropathy, which affects the hands and/or feet bilaterally; it is characterized by loss of sensation, abnormal sensations, pain, and paresthesias. (DM)

228. Correct answer – A. St. John's wort can decrease the antidiabetic effect of medication (for example, raise blood glucose). Other listed supplements have the opposite effect. (DA)

229. Correct answer – C. Manifestations of DKA include poor skin turgor, dry mucous membrances, tachycardia, othostatic hypotension, and Kussmaul respirations (rapid, deep breathing associated with dyspnea). (DD)

230. Correct answer – A. The onset for rapid-acting insulin is 15 minutes after injection; it peaks at 1 to 1.5 hours and lasts 3 to 4.5 hours. Short-acting insulin has an onset of 30 minutes. (DA)

231. Correct answer – C. Sulfonylureas, such as glyburide, increase insulin secretion. Glucosidase inhibitors, such as acarbose (Precose®), slow absorption of carbohydrates. (DT)

232. Correct answer – D. Lantus does not peak; it offers a 24-hour release for blood glucose control with one injection a day. (DT)

233. Correct answer – A. Lantus should never be mixed with other insulins because it will lose its effectiveness and affect blood glucose control. Lantus is clear and should be discarded 28 to 30 days after opening.

The same syringe should not be used for Lantus and other insulins. (DT)

234. Correct answer – C. Conditions that may cause secondary diabetes include hyperthyroidism and Cushing syndrome. Hypopituitarism, Hashimoto's thyroiditis, and Addison's disease can all lead to a hypoglycemic state. (DD)

235. Correct answer – A. The high blood glucose levels of HHNS increase serum osmolality and can produce severe neurologic manifestations such as somnolence, coma, seizures, hemiparesis, and aphasia. Arterial pH in HHNS is >7.3, and the patient tends to exhibit tachycardia and polyuria.

236. Correct answer – A. The highest incidence of diabetes mellitus is among Native Americans, 15% of whom are treated for the disease. Complications from diabetes mellitus are also the major causes of death in most Native American populations. (DD)

237. Correct answer – B. Insulin resistance syndrome is also know as cardiovascular dysmetabolic syndrome because of the cluster of abnormalities that greatly increase the risk for cardiovascular disease, elevated insulin levels, high levels of high-density lipoprotein (HDL), increased levels of low-density lipoprotein (LDL), and hypertension. (DM)

238. Correct answer – C. Rapid-acting insulin is considered to be the type that best mimics natural insulin secretion in response to meal. (DA)

239. Correct answer – B. Patients receiving long-term corticosteroids are likely to experience increased insulin resistance and gluconeogenesis. The other choices do not contribute to the development of HHNS. (DD)

240. Correct answer – A. The action of sulfonylureas is to increase insulin secretion. For a patient receiving combination therapy, skipping meals or snacks can trigger a hypoglycemic episode. (DM)

241. Correct answer – D. Risk factors for the development of diabetic

nephropathy include hypertension, smoking, and chronic hyperglycemia. (DT)

242. Correct answer – C. An A1C (also known as glycated hemoglobin or HbA1c) test provides a picture of the patient's average blood glucose control for the past 2 to 3 months. The results give a good idea of how well the diabetes treatment plan is working. (DM)

243. Correct answer – D. The insulin pump is programmed to deliver a continuous infusion of short-acting insulin 24 hours a day (basal rate). (DA)

References

Adams, H.P., del Zoppo, G., Alberts, M.J., Bhatt, D.L., Brass, L., Furlan, A., et al. (2007). Guidelines for the early management of adults with ischemic stroke. A guideline from the American Heart Association/American Stroke Association Stroke Council, Clinical Cardiology Council, Cardiovascular Radiology and Intervention Council, and the Atherosclerotic Peripheral Vascular Disease and Quality of Care Outcomes in Research Interdisciplinary Working Groups. *Stroke, 38*,1655.

American Heart Association. (2005). *American Heart Association guidelines for cardiopulmonary resuscitation and emergency cardiovascular care.* Retrieved December 27, 2007, from http://circ.ahajournals.org/cgi/content/full/112/24_suppl/IV-19

Black, J.M., & Hawks, J.H. (2004). *Medical-surgical nursing: Clinical management for positive outcomes* (7th ed.). Philadelphia: W.B. Saunders.

Blackbourne, L.H. (2003). *Advanced surgical recall.* Philadelphia: Lippincott, Williams & Wilkins.

Brozenac, S.A., & Russell, S.S. (2004). *Core curriculum for medical-surgical nursing* (3rd ed.). Pitman, NJ: Academy of Medical-Surgical Nurses.

Bunting-Perry, L.K. (2006).Palliative care in Parkinson's disease: Implications for neuroscience nursing. *Journal of Neuroscience Nursing, 38*(2),106-113.

Centers for Disease Control and Prevention. (2005). *Hepatitis B – CDC fact sheet.* Retrieved December 23, 2007, from http://www.cdc.gov/std/hepatitis/STDFact-Hepatitis-B.htm#Howspread

Centers for Disease Control and Prevention. (2007). *Mantoux tuberculosis skin test facilitator guide.* Retrieved December 23, 2007, from http://www.cdc.gov/tb/pubs/Mantoux/part2.htm

Cystic Fibrosis Foundation. (2006). *Nutrition: Bone health and cystic fibrosis.* Retrieved December 23, 2007, from http://www.cff.org/UploadedFiles/treatments/Therapies/Nutrition/BoneHealth/Nutrition%20%20Bone%20Health%20and%20Cystic%20Fibrosis.pdf

Durbin, C.G., Jr. (2005). Early complications of tracheostomy. *Respiratory Care, 50*(4), 511-515.

Holland, N.J., & Madonna, M. (2005). Nursing grand rounds: Multiple sclerosis. *Journal of Neuroscience Nursing, 37*(1), 15-19.

Huether, S., & McCance, K. (2004). *Understanding pathophysiology.* (3rd ed.). St. Louis: Mosby.

Ignatavicius, D., & Bayne, M.V. (2002). *Medical-surgical nursing: A nursing process approach* (4th ed., p. 783-787). Philadelphia: W.B. Saunders.

Ignatavicius, D.D., & Workman, M.L. (Eds.) (2005). *Medical-surgical nursing: Critical thinking for collaborative care* (5th ed.). Philadelphia: W.B. Saunders.

Lackey, S. (2006). Suppressing the scourge of AMI. *Nursing2006, 36*(5), 37-41.

Leeuwen, A., Kranpitz, T., & Smith, L. (2006). *Laboratory and diagnostic tests with nursing implications.* Philadelphia: FA Davis.

Lewis, S., Heitkemper, M., Dirksen, S.R., O'Brien, P.G., & Bucher, L. (2007*). Medical-surgical nursing: Assessment and management of clinical problems* (7th ed.). St. Louis: Mosby.

Maher, A.B., Salmond, S.W., & Pellino, T.A. (Eds.) (2002). *Orthopaedic nursing* (3rd ed.). Philadelphia: W.B. Saunders.

Matura, L., & Mengo, P. (2003). Guidelines for diagnosis and management of unstable angina and non-ST-segment elevation myocardial infarction. *Internet Journal of Advanced Nursing Practice, 6*(1), 1-14.

Morton, P., Fontaine, D., Hudak, C., & Gallo, B. (2005). *Critical care nursing: A holistic approach* (8th ed.). Philadelphia: Lippincott, Williams & Wilkins.

Mosher, C.M. (Ed.) (2004). *An introduction to orthopaedic nursing* (3rd ed.). Chicago: National Association of Orthopaedic Nurses.

National Association of Orthopaedic Nurses. (2007). *Core curriculum for orthopaedic nursing* (6th ed.). Chicago: Author.

Newswanger , D.L., & Warren, C.R. (2004). Guillain-Barré syndrome. *American Family Physician, 69*(10), 2405-2410.

Perry, A.G., & Potter, P.A. (2005). *Clinical nursing skills and techniques* (6th ed.). St. Louis, MO: Mosby.

Price, S., & Wilson, L. (2003). *Pathophysiology: Clinical concepts of disease processes* (6th ed.). St. Louis, MO: Mosby.

Robinson, K., Dennison, A., Roalf, D., Noorigian, J., Cianci, H., Bunting-Perry, L., et al. (2005). Falling risk factors in Parkinson´s disease. *NeuroRehabilitation, 20*(3),169-182.

Smeltzer, S., & Bare, B. (2004). *Brunner & Suddarth's textbook of medical-surgical nursing* (10th ed.). Philadelphia: Lippincott, Williams & Wilkins.

The Merck Manual. (2006a). Hepatic encephalopathy. Retrieved December 23, 2007, from http://www.merck.com/mmhe/sec10/ch135/ch135f.html

The Merck Manual. (2006b). Portal hypertension. Retrieved December 23, 2007, from https://www.merck.com/mmhe/sec10/ch135/ch135d.html

Turkoski, B., Lance, B., & Bonfiglio, M. (2006). *Drug information handbook for nursing.* (8th ed.). Hudson, OH: Lexi-Comp.

Wilson, B., Shannon, M., & Stang, C. (2004). *Nurse's drug guide 2004.* Upper Saddle River, NJ: Prentice Hall.

Medical-Surgical Nursing Review Questions Answer Sheet (#1-123)

1.	A	B	C	D	42.	A	B	C	D	83.	A	B	C	D
2.	A	B	C	D	43.	A	B	C	D	84.	A	B	C	D
3.	A	B	C	D	44.	A	B	C	D	85.	A	B	C	D
4.	A	B	C	D	45.	A	B	C	D	86.	A	B	C	D
5.	A	B	C	D	46.	A	B	C	D	87.	A	B	C	D
6.	A	B	C	D	47.	A	B	C	D	88.	A	B	C	D
7.	A	B	C	D	48.	A	B	C	D	89.	A	B	C	D
8.	A	B	C	D	49.	A	B	C	D	90.	A	B	C	D
9.	A	B	C	D	50.	A	B	C	D	91.	A	B	C	D
10.	A	B	C	D	51.	A	B	C	D	92.	A	B	C	D
11.	A	B	C	D	52.	A	B	C	D	93.	A	B	C	D
12.	A	B	C	D	53.	A	B	C	D	94.	A	B	C	D
13.	A	B	C	D	54.	A	B	C	D	95.	A	B	C	D
14.	A	B	C	D	55.	A	B	C	D	96.	A	B	C	D
15.	A	B	C	D	56.	A	B	C	D	97.	A	B	C	D
16.	A	B	C	D	57.	A	B	C	D	98.	A	B	C	D
17.	A	B	C	D	58.	A	B	C	D	99.	A	B	C	D
18.	A	B	C	D	59.	A	B	C	D	100.	A	B	C	D
19.	A	B	C	D	60.	A	B	C	D	101.	A	B	C	D
20.	A	B	C	D	61.	A	B	C	D	102.	A	B	C	D
21.	A	B	C	D	62.	A	B	C	D	103.	A	B	C	D
22.	A	B	C	D	63.	A	B	C	D	104.	A	B	C	D
23.	A	B	C	D	64.	A	B	C	D	105.	A	B	C	D
24.	A	B	C	D	65.	A	B	C	D	106.	A	B	C	D
25.	A	B	C	D	66.	A	B	C	D	107.	A	B	C	D
26.	A	B	C	D	67.	A	B	C	D	108.	A	B	C	D
27.	A	B	C	D	68.	A	B	C	D	109.	A	B	C	D
28.	A	B	C	D	69.	A	B	C	D	110.	A	B	C	D
29.	A	B	C	D	70.	A	B	C	D	111.	A	B	C	D
30.	A	B	C	D	71.	A	B	C	D	112.	A	B	C	D
31.	A	B	C	D	72.	A	B	C	D	113	A	B	C	D
32.	A	B	C	D	73.	A	B	C	D	114.	A	B	C	D
33.	A	B	C	D	74.	A	B	C	D	115.	A	B	C	D
34.	A	B	C	D	75.	A	B	C	D	116.	A	B	C	D
35.	A	B	C	D	76.	A	B	C	D	117.	A	B	C	D
36.	A	B	C	D	77.	A	B	C	D	118.	A	B	C	D
37.	A	B	C	D	78.	A	B	C	D	119.	A	B	C	D
38.	A	B	C	D	79.	A	B	C	D	120.	A	B	C	D
39.	A	B	C	D	80.	A	B	C	D	121.	A	B	C	D
40.	A	B	C	D	81.	A	B	C	D	122.	A	B	C	D
41.	A	B	C	D	82.	A	B	C	D	123.	A	B	C	D

124.	A	B	C	D	165.	A	B	C	D	206.	A	B	C	D
125.	A	B	C	D	166.	A	B	C	D	207.	A	B	C	D
126.	A	B	C	D	167.	A	B	C	D	208.	A	B	C	D
127.	A	B	C	D	168.	A	B	C	D	209.	A	B	C	D
128.	A	B	C	D	169.	A	B	C	D	210.	A	B	C	D
129.	A	B	C	D	170.	A	B	C	D	211.	A	B	C	D
130.	A	B	C	D	171.	A	B	C	D	212.	A	B	C	D
131.	A	B	C	D	272.	A	B	C	D	213.	A	B	C	D
232.	A	B	C	D	173.	A	B	C	D	214.	A	B	C	D
133.	A	B	C	D	174.	A	B	C	D	215.	A	B	C	D
134.	A	B	C	D	175.	A	B	C	D	216.	A	B	C	D
135.	A	B	C	D	176.	A	B	C	D	217.	A	B	C	D
136.	A	B	C	D	177.	A	B	C	D	218.	A	B	C	D
137.	A	B	C	D	178.	A	B	C	D	219.	A	B	C	D
138.	A	B	C	D	179.	A	B	C	D	220.	A	B	C	D
139.	A	B	C	D	180.	A	B	C	D	221.	A	B	C	D
140.	A	B	C	D	181.	A	B	C	D	222.	A	B	C	D
141.	A	B	C	D	182.	A	B	C	D	223	A	B	C	D
142.	A	B	C	D	183.	A	B	C	D	224.	A	B	C	D
143.	A	B	C	D	184.	A	B	C	D	225.	A	B	C	D
144.	A	B	C	D	185.	A	B	C	D	226.	A	B	C	D
145.	A	B	C	D	186.	A	B	C	D	227.	A	B	C	D
146.	A	B	C	D	187.	A	B	C	D	228.	A	B	C	D
147.	A	B	C	D	188.	A	B	C	D	229.	A	B	C	D
148.	A	B	C	D	189.	A	B	C	D	230.	A	B	C	D
149.	A	B	C	D	190.	A	B	C	D	231.	A	B	C	D
150.	A	B	C	D	191.	A	B	C	D	232.	A	B	C	D
151.	A	B	C	D	192.	A	B	C	D	233.	A	B	C	D
252.	A	B	C	D	193.	A	B	C	D	234.	A	B	C	D
153.	A	B	C	D	194.	A	B	C	D	235.	A	B	C	D
154.	A	B	C	D	195.	A	B	C	D	236.	A	B	C	D
155.	A	B	C	D	196.	A	B	C	D	237.	A	B	C	D
156.	A	B	C	D	197.	A	B	C	D	138.	A	B	C	D
157.	A	B	C	D	198.	A	B	C	D	239.	A	B	C	D
158.	A	B	C	D	199.	A	B	C	D	240.	A	B	C	D
159.	A	B	C	D	200.	A	B	C	D	241.	A	B	C	D
160.	A	B	C	D	201.	A	B	C	D	242.	A	B	C	D
161.	A	B	C	D	202.	A	B	C	D	243.	A	B	C	D
162.	A	B	C	D	203.	A	B	C	D					
163.	A	B	C	D	204.	A	B	C	D					
164.	A	B	C	D	205.	A	B	C	D					

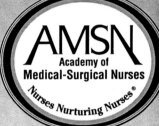

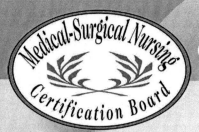

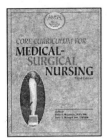
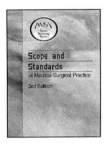
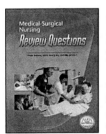
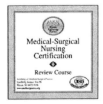
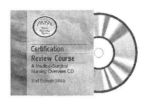
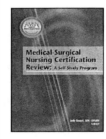

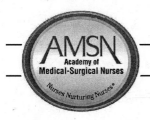

The Academy of Medical-Surgical Nurses

History

It is likely that the idea of adult health nursing as a specialty practice area in nursing was born in the mid-19th century when Florence Nightingale took 38 women to the Crimea to care for the sick and dying British solders in 1856. Not long after that, American men and women took on the same burden during the Civil War. While not yet recognized as a specialty group, adults with a gamut of physiologic needs were the specific concern of these caregivers. Throughout the history of organized nursing that followed these two national catastrophes, the classification of adult patients into medical and/or surgical categories has been prevalent.

A criterion for an established profession is the organization of a specialty group that governs standards of practice and ethical codes and monitors quality among the membership. In nursing, the American Nurses Association (ANA) and the National League for Nursing (NLN) have acted in this capacity since the turn of the century. Beginning in 1954 with the establishment of the Association of Operating Room Nurses (AORN), specialty groups formed to meet the specific needs of those working with a particular client population. In 1991, recognizing the lack of a national organization to act as a forum for medical-surgical nurses, Cecelia Grindel and Alice Poyss established the groundwork for the Academy of Medical-Surgical Nurses (AMSN). AMSN was chartered in Philadelphia in October 1991.

Mission

The Academy of Medical-Surgical Nurses enhances the knowledge, skills, and professionalism of medical-surgical/adult health nurses in all practice settings.

Vision

The medical-surgical/adult health nurse is a valued health care professional and a vital part of the health care continuum committed to leadership, quality care and advocacy for patients, their families, and the communities in which they live and work.

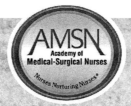

Academy of Medical-Surgical Nurses
East Holly Avenue/Box 56, Pitman, New Jersey 08071-0056
Phone: 856-256-2323
Toll-Free: 866-877-AMSN (2676)
Fax: 856-589-7463
Email: amsn@ajj.com
Web site: www.medsurgnurse.org